"*The 9 Pillars of Resilience* offers a deep and welcomed exploration of the universal laws of life, guiding readers through the intricate relationship between mind, body, and spirit. It presents actionable insights for overcoming unconscious barriers and optimizing personal energy. With a blend of ancient wisdom and modern science, Dr. Sideroff masterfully equips you with the tools for achieving greater happiness, health, and success, making this an essential read for anyone seeking to navigate life's complexities with grace and effectiveness."

—**David Perlmutter, MD, #1** *New York Times*
bestselling author of *Grain Brain* **and** *Drop Acid*

"This is a terrific book. I love *The 9 Pillars of Resilience*, and feel it is a true Bible for living in balance and spirituality. Dr. Stephen Sideroff has created a marvelous guide to finding and staying on the Path through systematic exercises and the contemporary image of the 'primitive Gestalt.' The book is a masterful blending of empirical research results with the personal journey in a delightful, clear and engaging structure to accompany the reader in their growth toward balance, deeper meaning, and the world beyond."

—**Ron Doctor, PhD, clinical psychologist, author,**
and board-certified expert in trauma

"Optimal health, wellness and longevity include the effective tackling of mental and emotional challenges and life's stresses. Just as food is medicine, Dr. Sideroff's insightful and comprehensive approach to resilience presents the equivalent mental and emotional medicine to help the body function at its best. His easy-to-follow and effective techniques support the development of optimal resilience to complement what we choose to eat. Presented as a step-by-step program, with solutions that build mental clarity, *The 9 Pillars of Resilience* offers practical, yet deeply transformative processes for both health and success."

—**Mark Hyman, MD, Pritzker Foundation chair in functional**
medicine at Cleveland Clinic Lerner College of Medicine

"Our research has shown that brain health and cognitive decline involve multiple interrelated factors. One of the most important is chronic stress, so I am grateful for information that can help patients cope better and minimize its impact. That's why I was so pleased to read Dr. Stephen Sideroff's excellent book, *The 9 Pillars of Resilience*, which clearly demonstrates the connection between mind and body, providing the ultimate guide for developing lifelong habits of adaptability and mental balance to take life stresses in stride and restore nervous system health. The book describes what Dr. Sideroff calls 'the Path' which is a creative blueprint to help us all stay committed to behavioral and mental changes to break free of outdated habits. It's filled with practical advice and actionable takeaways. It is an excellent book for our times, and is indispensable for anyone struggling with stress or unwanted physical symptoms. I highly recommend Dr. Sideroff's *The 9 Pillars of Resilience*."

—**Dale Bredesen, MD, author of the** *New York*
Times **bestseller** *The End of Alzheimer's*

"An extraordinary blueprint for resilience. Dr. Sideroff has an incredible ability to distill complex processes into an easy to follow pathway toward building resilience. I truly feel something profound shifting in me after working through *The 9 Pillars*. Thank you for so eloquently putting decades of wisdom into this book. Highly recommend!"

—**Sarah Abedi, MD, emergency medicine physician
and host of the *Hidden Body Podcast***

"My life has been devoted to anti-aging and life extension. If you can slow aging, you can prevent illness. Dr. Sideroff addresses one of the most important factors that speeds up aging and thus the development of symptoms. I'm impressed with Dr. Sideroff's comprehensive and innovative model of resilience. But what makes his book most valuable is the step-by-step approach that I believe anyone can follow to gain new coping skills and live life with greater calmness and health. Anyone overwhelmed by stress should get this book."

—**Bill Faloon, founder of Life Extension**

"Beautifully written, combining the latest scientific insights about the brain's mechanisms to respond to perturbations with practical lessons and assignments, Dr. Sideroff's book provides a badly needed resource for many people trying to maneuver through a world packed with challenges that evolution has not equipped us well to cope with effectively. This book is a must read for people that feel overwhelmed psychologically, or even worse, that are suffering from physical symptoms related to allostatic load."

—**Emeran A. Mayer, MD, executive director of the G. Oppenheimer
Center for Neurobiology of Stress and Resilience**

"As a cardiologist, I'm always looking for healthier lifestyle modifications that my patients can benefit from. This is a great book for anyone struggling with all the stresses in their lives, or with nagging physical symptoms. I highly recommend *The 9 Pillars of Resilience*. My friend and colleague, Dr. Sideroff, has created a comprehensive and easy to follow model and methodology to develop resilience. There are many books on this subject. What makes this book stand out is how well Stephen has laid out an approach that takes you by the hand and keeps you on the Path. This book will help you stay focused on overcoming old habits and developing a new and effective way of living each day with balance and joy. Get *The 9 Pillars of Resilience*, put it next to your bed, and read a few pages every day. It will change your life."

—**Joel Kahn, MD, Director of the Kahn Center for Cardiac Longevity**

"Dr. Stephen Sideroff's book, *The 9 Pillars of Resilience*, is a transformative guide that bridges the gap between scientific research and practical application. Through his insightful exploration of resilience, Dr. Sideroff offers readers a comprehensive road map to not only withstand the challenges of life but to thrive amidst them. Dr. Sideroff's writing is both accessible and profound, making complex concepts easily understandable and, more importantly, actionable. I wholeheartedly recommend *The 9 Pillars of Resilience* to anyone seeking to navigate life's challenges with grace, strength, and vitality."

—**Karol Darsa, PsyD, executive director at Reconnect Integrative Trauma Treatment Center**

"*The 9 Pillars of Resilience* is an insightful book that provides the reader with practical, implementable strategies to manage stress and its negative impact on our health, lives, and relationships. The best part of this book is the commitment of only five minutes a day to effect long term change. As a physician, the recognition of the 'autonomic dysregulation syndrome' and its effect on our physical well-being is evident but modifying our maladaptive behaviors is never easy. The Path of Resilience Questionnaire allows the readers to self-assess their profile on the 9 Pillars of Resilience identified by Dr. Sideroff. Through the exercises for each day of the year, action steps, journaling and reflection, Dr. Sideroff guides the reader toward the 9 Pillars of Resilience and all the benefits of better stress management."

—**Tenaz Kermani, MD, founder and director of UCLA's multidisciplinary vasculitis program and professor of rheumatology at UCLA's Geffen School of Medicine**

"*The 9 Pillars of Resilience* artfully distills Stephen Sideroff's vast knowledge of personal development, neuroscience, and self-regulation arts. I love 'The Path' and the idea of tools for moving along the path and returning to it when you discover you are off your life's path. His 9 Pillars of Resilience enable you to assess yourself and self-regulate. Engagingly written, *The 9 Pillars of Resilience* is a comprehensive guide for you along your path."

—**Eleanor Criswell, EdD, clinical psychologist, author of *Biofeedback and Somatics*, and past president of the International Society of Yoga Therapists**

"Dr. Sideroff brings together the science of physiology and the wisdom of transformational psychology for the cultivation of mental and emotional adaptability. Stephen is a gifted writer who manages to take complex ideas and present them in an approachable manner, guiding the reader on a step-by-step path of personal growth. In my medical practice I identify patients' blockages to physical, emotional and mental resilience. Where I have had methods of balancing physiologic adaptability, I had not found the right material to support emotional and mental balance—until now. I will recommend *The Path* to my patients and students alike."

—**Kamyar M. Hedayat, MD, president of the American Society of Endobiogenic Medicine and Integrative Physiology and medical director at Full Spectrum Health: An Endobiogeny Medical Clinic**

"In *The 9 Pillars of Resilience*, Stephen Sideroff's extensive experience is evident as he has created a powerful approach to mastering life's stresses that are overwhelming so many of us. This is an eminently readable book that anticipates people's resistance to change, and uses the concept of The Path in a step-by-step process that anyone can access to achieve transformation and happiness in their lives."

—**Dr. Lynda Thompson, executive director of the ADD Centre, Ltd.**

"*The 9 Pillars of Resilience* is more than just a book; it's a beacon of hope for those navigating life's challenges. As someone who works with people grappling with stress, I can confidently say that this book is a game changer. The step-by-step approach is a much needed well-lit path. The author's ability to break down complex concepts into actionable steps is commendable. From emotional intelligence to physical well-being, each of the nine pillars contributes to resilience. Reading this book feels like having a compassionate mentor by your side. If you're ready to embark on a transformative journey—one that nourishes your mind, body, and spirit—pick up this book today."

—**Dr. Heather Sandison, ND, author of *Reversing Alzheimer's***

"I have had the privilege of knowing Dr. Stephen Sideroff for many years, and I am continually inspired by his dedication to empowering individuals to lead fulfilling and resilient lives. As Dr. Sideroff completes yet another groundbreaking book on the foundations of resilience, I am compelled to share my enthusiastic endorsement of his work. Dr. Sideroff's unique blend of scientific expertise, coupled with his wealth of life experience, sets him apart as a leading authority in the field of resilience. His commitment to rigorous research ensures that his insights are not only profound but also firmly grounded in empirical evidence. What truly sets Dr. Sideroff apart, however, is his compassionate heart and genuine desire to make a positive difference in the world. He approaches his work with a rare combination of intellect and empathy, creating a safe and supportive space for individuals to explore and cultivate their resilience. Through his writing, Dr. Sideroff offers practical guidance and invaluable wisdom for those seeking to create a wonderful life on multiple levels. His book promises to be an indispensable resource for anyone navigating life's challenges and striving to unlock their full potential. I wholeheartedly recommend Dr. Stephen Sideroff and his forthcoming book to anyone interested in harnessing the power of resilience to lead a more fulfilling and meaningful life. His insights have the potential to transform lives, and I am grateful for the opportunity to bear witness to his impactful work."

—**Dr. Allen Darbonne, director of the University Center for Optimal Relationships & Neurofeedback**

THE 9 PILLARS OF RESILIENCE

The Proven Path to Master Stress,
Slow Aging, and Increase Vitality

Dr. Stephen I. Sideroff

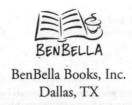

BenBella Books, Inc.
Dallas, TX

BenBella Books, Inc.
10440 N. Central Expressway
Suite 800
Dallas, TX 75231
benbellabooks.com
Send feedback to feedback@benbellabooks.com

BenBella is a federally registered trademark.

Printed in the United States of America
10 9 8 7 6 5 4 3 2 1

Library of Congress Control Number: 2023058371
ISBN 9781637745557 (hardcover)
ISBN 9781637745564 (electronic)

Copyediting by Scott Calamar
Proofreading by Jenny Bridges and Ashley Casteel
Text design and composition by PerfecType, Nashville, TN
Cover design by Brigid Pearson
Printed by Lake Book Manufacturing

To my grandmother Mini and grandfather Sam Kessler
To my mother, Ruth, and father, Jerry
And to my wife, Freda
All have contributed greatly to my resilience and success

CONTENTS

FOREWORD

I have followed the work of my friend and colleague Stephen Sideroff for a number of years. Stephen and I share a passion for facilitating the healing process and restoring the body's natural ability to recover inner balance. Stephen's model for achieving resilience, The Path, goes a long way toward identifying the factors that contribute to trauma and stress, and it offers effective ways to relieve them. I was impressed by Stephen's ability to distill his entire process into just one question: "Am I on or off The Path?"—and his promise that, even if you stumble off The Path, you can always find your way back to it. In addition, his resilience assessment tool helps readers quickly identify areas of strength and those areas they need to work on as they journey along The Path.

In my work, Somatic Experiencing, I talk about unfreezing from traumatic events. Stephen refers to the shifting from a pattern that's frozen by one's attachment to his or her primitive Gestalt, a childhood blueprint, an engram that unconsciously guides all our behaviors—creating a gravitational pull that's hard to break out of. Stephen takes readers by the hand, guiding them through a step-by-step process designed to optimize the way they react to stress and increase their ability to adapt and handle challenging circumstances. He presents a way to overcome the personal blocks that interfere with the average individual's ability to achieve success. Stephen has developed these exercises and methodology based on a lifetime of research, lessons gleaned from his clinical practice, and the training of other clinicians.

Stephen does a great job of anticipating the difficulties and resistance that each reader will bring to the process of growth. Reading his book, I was able to appreciate the unique perspective he brings to bear in his efforts to help the reader achieve resilience and, ultimately, success along life's "Path." I encourage you to take this book and these exercises to heart. Those who follow the lessons laid out here can lead a life of optimal health, success, and happiness, even under difficult circumstances.

Peter Levine, PhD
Founder of Somatic Experiencing
Bestselling author of *Waking the Tiger, Healing Trauma,* and *In an Unspoken Voice: How the Body Releases Trauma and Restores Goodness*
Lyons, Colorado

PREFACE

When I began presenting peak performance workshops for executives in 1980, I recognized that one of the most important ingredients to success was learning the concept of flow and being in the zone. These concepts are most frequently mentioned in relation to sports, but they define peak performance in all areas. They refer to a way of functioning in which everything is working together, in alignment. When you are in the zone, you don't have to think about what you are doing; you just do it, as the Nike trademark says.

It became evident to me that one common denominator for people in the zone or in flow was adaptability. "Adaptability" refers to the ability to learn from experience, continually take in new information, and adjust your thinking and behavior to accommodate new lessons of life. Flexible and aware, these peak performers did not get stuck on any one particular way of thinking or acting. Interestingly, these same people were very good at managing the inevitable stresses that accompanied their success.

This led to my own research into successful living. I saw many people who were able to make a lot of money or show good results in their company's bottom line but whom I would not consider peak performers. Many of them were referred to me by physicians to address their high blood pressure, headaches, or sleepless nights. Others would find their way to my doorstep for help with conflict-ridden relationships or simply dissatisfaction or unhappiness with their lives. Their performance in business did not translate into peak performance in life.

At the same time, I was working with another group of clients who were feeling stuck in their lives. Despite all their hard work, they never seemed to break through to another level. They got bogged down or overwhelmed by the details of their lives or distracted by ongoing conflicts.

The commonality between these two populations was their difficulty in learning from their mistakes or recognizing how their thinking and attitude interfered with their success. Their thinking was rigid, and they had many blind spots—areas off-limits to their awareness. Weaknesses remained weaknesses. Nowhere was this more evident than in how these clients handled stress.

Many refer to resilience as the ability to bounce back after a stressful experience. But in my definition of resilience, there is more to the process than simply bouncing back. I refer to it as "bouncing forward." This is where the stressful experience triggers new adaptive learning, resulting in becoming a better version of yourself with each life challenge you face. This more expansive definition of resilience shows why I find it important to embrace challenges rather than shrinking from them or engaging reluctantly. Frozen adaptability is the hallmark of being stuck in the lessons of childhood, what I term, and will be discussing, your "primitive Gestalt patterns."

In my study of these populations, I realized that stress and how effectively one handles stress are primary modulators of quality of life and success in life. Stress can accentuate a person's weaknesses, lead to physical and emotional symptoms, and cause a breakdown in various aspects of one's life. Mastering stress is the hallmark of adaptability and a consistent marker of overall life success. Thus, within my program, I make a distinction between business success and life success (although life success can incorporate business success). I refer to this broader and richer concept, sought by executives and others who come to me, as "Resilient Success."

No one is immune to the consequences and even the seduction of stress. The more you try to achieve, the more stress you face. Those who don't have enough money work harder to make ends meet or worry that they won't make ends meet. However, many people who are well-off somehow keep the demands of their lives a bit greater than either the time or resources available to meet those demands.

I remember one executive who had come upon bad times. Business projects weren't panning out, and he found himself in financial difficulty. To rectify the situation, he began new projects. At the same time, he continued to work on old projects that were problematic. All in all, his life was filled with stressful experiences. Week after week we addressed his decision-making, problem-solving, and goal setting. Slowly but surely, more and more of his life was getting under control. His ship was righting itself, the last piece of difficulty was being addressed, and he was preparing to breathe a sigh of relief. The following week, he entered my office with a new set of stressful problems. Sadly, this scenario is not an isolated example.

I fully expected participants in my workshops to grasp the straightforward ways to reduce stress and implement more effective coping mechanisms. After all, even my most "successful" clients reported growing numbers of symptoms related to the fast pace of their lives. Instead, over the years I encountered more and more obstacles to success—and to awareness. My clients and workshop participants found more and more creative ways to continually activate their stress response, to be vigilant and to worry, even when they could have been relaxing. This occurred despite evidence that quality and effectiveness in their lives were directly impacted by their maladaptive behavior.

Were all these people coming to see me simply caught up in fortune? Or was I observing a more universal process—with th' ents just the extreme cases?

I began studying and cataloging this all-too-common resistance to reducing stress. Consequences included distraction, loss of focus, fatigue, forgetfulness, and mistakes. (Think of the photos you've seen of our recent presidents—photos taken at the start of their presidency and photos taken when they are leaving office. That's stress and aging before our very eyes!)

This was an eye-opener! Despite all the ravages of stress—and a growing accumulation of research demonstrates the destructive impact of stress—people continually engage in behaviors that strain their coping resources and cause widespread physical and emotional destruction. I encountered smart people who were having difficulty engaging in adaptive behaviors. Finally, about fifteen years ago, in response to people's harmful behavior, I developed a new direction for my work, one that focused on the importance of adaptability.

Our stress response is an evolutionary adaptive mechanism. It prepares us for danger. It saves our lives. Instinctually, we are reluctant to curb that response. My research, however, revealed a large maladaptive component to being in almost continual stress alert. Furthermore, this unhealthy pattern carries over into other areas of thinking and performance.

CHILDHOOD PATTERNS AND ADAPTABILITY

We are intimately attached to patterns developed during childhood. The brain develops and adapts to this earliest learning. What must be kept in mind is that first learning is survival learning—thus, attachment to these lessons holds the highest level of importance and strength. This survival-level importance is coded into our lessons of how the world works and who we are, rendering adaptation to newer information more difficult. In other words, childhood development can interfere with healthy adult adaptation! We are given the chart of the territory of life and ourselves but not the keys to make healthy changes to the chart. I will expand upon this concept later, when I describe what I have termed "primitive Gestalts," which are these learned and fixed childhood "neurobiological" patterns.

In working with clients to address this inherent obstacle, I needed an approach that didn't trigger resistance with every turn. It's like the patient who goes to the doctor to relieve a symptom or illness, and the doctor says, "Sir, you have to get to bed earlier, you have to stop smoking, you have to exercise more, stop drinking, and you have to lose weight." And the patient leaves the office saying, "I have to get another doctor." That's when I wrote my first article: "Resilience: a Unimotivational Approach to Stress and Success."

I didn't realize at first that all the disparate pieces I was working on were fitting into a model of resilience. What I developed was not a program of restrictions; instead, it's all about optimal functioning, making the best choices and—above all—mastering the use of personal energy. Yes, "personal energy," the organismic resources that are available to you.

Ultimately, this book presents a comprehensive, logical, and organized integration of optimal functioning that restores and maintains personal energy. It serves as a blueprint and guidance device for creating greater adaptability. Furthermore, it is designed to work at the deepest levels. After all, the source of personal energy is derived from your deepest self.

There have been many self-help approaches to peak performance as well as coping with stress. However, the "I" that works this program is embedded in your personal neurobiobehavioral patterns (this simply means how your brain got wired)—what I have termed your "primitive Gestalts." In other words, as you read this, you have a bias created by childhood lessons that may not serve you. Other programs don't address the undermining nature of these unconscious beliefs, emotions, or thinking. From the start, most books work the surface of behavior.

Within the pages of this book, you will be introduced to a model of Resilient Success I have developed after years of studying optimal functioning and the mastery, rather than the control, of stress. It is about learning to bounce forward rather than bouncing back. My model of resilience identifies nine comprehensive components of being healthy, happy, and successful. This means for the best health, for the ability to reach your goals, for the greatest and deepest sense of happiness, as well as the opportunity to slow down the aging process. Oh, and one more thing: to have the most positive and impactful effect on the world! Each pillar contributes to a foundation of development that can literally restructure your brain based on its optimal functioning.

In all my previous work, my approach has been to meet you, the reader, listener, or trainee, where you are right now, and to help support and bring you forward. This book continues this tradition. As noted, I realized from my years of clinical experience that old patterns die hard, and we continually engage in unconscious sabotage or distraction due to stresses and unconsciousness. Thus I have devised, in conjunction with my model, a step-by-step program for its implementation, which I refer to as "The Path."

Within these pages I invite you to follow, at your own speed, the steps on The Path. Step onto The Path, and I will show you that it is associated with success, defined any way you desire. If you make it your intention to walk The Path, it will result in your optimal performance and help you achieve all that you want.

CHAPTER 1

INTRODUCTION

THE LAWS OF LIFE

One of the greatest points of leverage I have when consulting or working with clients is my knowledge of what I refer to as the primary or "universal laws of life." This is not just my perspective; my position is grounded in a group of fundamental principles about how mind, body, and spirit operate.

One of these principles is that unconsciousness, or lack of awareness, will always interfere with the achievement of your goals, and it will create invisible obstacles and contradictory motivations in your life. Another basic principle is that any self-deprecating or self-abusive talk is never helpful and thus never OK. Another principle states that the level of organismic activation—how much concern you display and how much you mobilize to allay that concern—should correlate with the importance of the event.

I use these and additional laws of life to define a set of primary rules that help guide your behavior and measure your progress. For example, every time you respond to an event, you activate your body and expend your personal energy. Every time you experience stress in the form of danger, uncertainty, worry, or fear, your body activates in response. One of the hallmarks of resilience is optimal activation, which means activating precisely to the level required by the event. Clearly, you want to activate enough to successfully address the experience. But you don't want to overreact or expend too much energy. In addition, resilience is about returning to a ready state of calm focus after the activating event is over, rather than continuing the activation when it's no longer necessary.

Worrying or thinking too much about a problem causes tension that is not constructive. Similarly, when you are unable to let go of a difficult event and continue to be activated by it, you are wasting precious psychic energy. This overactivation, as you will learn, is the source of imbalance and potential burnout. Thus, the goal is to be able to optimize energy use. Now you might ask me, "But wait, what if there really is something to worry about, something bad that might happen?" Here is where true resilience comes in: Appropriate planning is definitely important, but once you do this planning, continuing to go over the same thoughts is what I refer to as worry, which is never helpful. Activating your nervous system and stress response when there isn't a constructive response to make (meaning when the response will not have a positive impact) is the prime example of wasted and even toxic energy.

Life is uncertain. Something is always happening somewhere that may change your life. As an example, we can look at the tragedy in Japan during the winter of 2011, when a major earthquake, followed by a giant tsunami, changed people's lives forever. The other reality of everyday life is that it's very, very complex. Uncertainty and complexity are triggers for your body's adaptive survival mechanism. Most people are not well prepared for adapting to this type of world; you never got the appropriate training. Remarkably, it's not something taught in school. I suspect that's because our very educators are subject to the same unconscious behavioral choices as the pupils they teach. In fact, the training most people receive is counterproductive—leaving you even less prepared than you would be without any training at all.

Typically, there are multiple choices surrounding every aspect of your life. Wouldn't it be helpful, wouldn't it be freeing, if there really was "The Path"—a guideline for always making the right choice in how to act and what perspective to take? That is the goal of this book: to show you The Path, how to get on it and stay on it.

Why did you buy this book? What are you looking for? No matter what, you can break it down into two parts: (1) to achieve your goals, and (2) to be as happy and healthy as possible in the process of achieving these goals. I find there are two groups who come to me for help: those who are experiencing physical or emotional pain resulting from ongoing imbalance and those who are doing OK but know they can be doing better, feeling healthier, or performing better.

The challenge and goal of this book is to find "The Path" for yourself. In addition, I hope to present information that motivates, encourages, and supports deep and significant change, and even transformation, in the following ways:

- Enhanced use and management of your personal energy, resulting in the greater availability of resources for important tasks
- Improved recovery after stress
- Increased focus and overall effectiveness
- Better relationship with yourself; less critical, less negative, more accepting
- Improved relationships with others: setting appropriate boundaries, making good relationship choices, being assertive in getting your needs met, and thwarting those who want to take from you or pull you down
- Less emotional reactivity

- Improved physical health and recovery from illness
- Better thinking patterns and better decision-making with fewer mistakes
- Greater flexibility and more satisfaction in life
- Increased ability to achieve goals
- And finally, greater happiness in your life

In order for these goals to be achieved, certain universal laws need to be learned and then followed, as noted earlier in this chapter. You can't fudge with these laws. And there are no shortcuts. For example, if you have lost some of your ability to relax, as manifested by sleep problems, frequent headaches, or illness, you need to retrain your body. That requires practicing some form of relaxation technique. Like any other learning or training process, practice makes perfect.

These are not rules I personally have invented. They are universal principles I uncovered after years of working with thousands of individuals. I have consistently found that when people disregard or are ignorant of these rules, they encounter more and greater problems that lead to crises. They experience more accidents in their lives, more unfulfilling relationships, and greater stress and illness. Let me emphasize here: These laws are not open to debate. Ignore them at your own risk and inevitable pain. Remember, you don't mess with Mother Nature!

FLOW AND THE LIFE FORCE

We are designed by nature to function effectively. Your body engages in literally thousands of functions from moment to moment to keep itself in balance. If your blood pressure becomes elevated, sensors in your blood vessels send signals to make adjustments that bring your blood pressure back down. If you are injured, resources are mobilized to heal the injury. With each demand placed on your body, processes are put into play to handle the demand. Fueling all these processes is your life energy or life force.

The concept of life force goes back many centuries. It forms the philosophical basis of many ancient traditions, including the Chinese notion of qi and the body's meridian system, as well as the yogi science of prana. Think of it as the flow of energy through and around the body.

For peak performance and resilience, you must master the concept of the life force. We don't have an unlimited amount. It is important to understand the principles that determine the efficient use of this force, as well as how it can be replenished. Without such awareness and by continuing many of your habitual patterns, you interfere with the flow of this life force. This will likely result in fatigue, illness, and less overall effectiveness in your life.

For most of us, this life force is used exclusively for survival. This was the default condition of our hunter-gatherer ancestors, and it did help them to survive . . . usually to the age of twenty or twenty-five. But for resilient success—meaning a long, healthy life—it is important to master the factors that contribute to the optimal utilization of this force and its regeneration. This requires a shift from an overwhelming focus on survival and stress to a balance between survival and creativity/adaptability. Throughout this book I will help you address this process by referring to "reaching inside" or opening to the deepest place inside yourself.

We actually start off in life set up for optimal adaptation and adjustment to our environment. The process is referred to as "homeostasis," the ability of the organism to achieve stability and always return to a place of balance. This process is designed to maintain the life force through continual renewal.

Ironically, it is adaptation to your childhood environment that is the major cause of your problems. Whatever is learned here about reward and punishment gets generalized to the world, locking you into a pattern with reduced ability to adapt.

Certain qualities help us be and stay in the flow while others keep us frozen. Below, I have presented the conditions that determine adaptability or being stuck:

Adaptability and optimal flow of the life force	Development of fixed patterns interfering with flow
Active—responsible for results in life	Passive—helpless about results in life
Open to new ways	Closed to new ways
Plasticity—available for change	Gravity—held back by the old
Positive attitude	Negative attitude
Receptive	Defensive
Flexible	Rigid
Internal locus of control	External locus of control
Self-guided	Guided by the rules of others
Why it's possible	Why it's difficult

GRASPING THE POSSIBLE

For many years, breaking the four-minute mile in track and field was thought to be impossible. And then one day in June 1954, Roger Bannister, an Australian, broke the four-minute mile with a time of 3 minutes, 59.4 seconds. The recognition of the possibility of this feat resulted in ten other runners breaking this barrier within one year of Bannister's triumph. In other words, the myth of its impossibility held runners back, and the reality of its possibility yielded numerous breakthroughs.

I want to help you believe that resilience and optimal functioning are possible. I want to show you that "The Path" will take you there and, most importantly, that it's within your grasp. That it's always just steps away. In other words, more than simply informing you and capturing your interest, I want this book to bridge the gap between what you learn and know, and what you believe and actually do.

Change involves a very basic yet difficult-to-achieve force. When I first began presenting seminars thirty years ago, I was excited about teaching people what they could do to reduce their stress, handle it better, and live a better life. Participants of my seminars and workshops attended because they were challenged and even overwhelmed by the demands of their lives and the symptoms they were experiencing. Yet, after listening to my program and leaving with enthusiasm about following through, six months down the road, they had fallen back into their old patterns.

Despite experiencing the consequences of too much stress, many people resist doing anything about it. Change is difficult, after all, no matter how motivated you are. This ordinarily difficult process is exacerbated by our specific resistance to dealing with stress and changing our habitual patterns. For the past twenty-five years, I have been researching and experimenting with ways to address one of the most primal forces known to humankind. I have described this force as each person's primitive Gestalt. It carries with it a gravitational pull, holding behaviors and thinking in place.

Primitive Gestalts are the neurobiobehavioral patterns established as the result of early survival learning. A more detailed discussion of primitive Gestalts will be found in chapter two. Briefly, primitive Gestalts (PG) are conceptualized as fixed patterns in the brain, and they exert a gravitational force on all our behaviors, perceptions, and thinking. This gravitational force makes fundamental change as difficult as it is for a rocket ship to leave the earth's gravitational pull or an electron to leave its orbit around the nucleus of the atom. This book— *The 9 Pillars of Resistance*—is the culmination of my research and experience helping thousands of people achieve this step in their lives.

Juxtaposed to the gravitational pull of your primitive Gestalts is the equally powerful neurobiological process of neuroplasticity. This is your brain's ability to rewire itself based on new learning. In fact, when you hold a new intention, such as a more supportive way of thinking about yourself, and are persistent with this intention, you actually create new nerve fibers and new connections. By reading or listening to the lessons of this book you are, in this moment, redesigning your brain and making it more resilient!

We can say that at the heart of Resilient Success is the ability to shift one's pattern and not be stuck in rigid thinking and behaving and excess emotional reactivity. Thus, part of the process of this book is to help you loosen the hold that your PG has on you—to block its "attractor state" quality and even to show you how it's no longer needed. Part of this process involves labeling some of your old thinking as "harmful."

As you move forward on The Path, together we will visualize a new attractor state, one that you personally create. The process of visualization is like planting the seeds for something new. By fully visualizing it—its qualities, its shape, why it's attractive, why it should be an attractor state—you will be watering those seeds, opening the doors of neuroplasticity, and beginning literally to guide the expression of your genes, your biological blueprint. You'll express them through the development of new nerve cells that enhance neural or brain connections. Those connections will become stronger, more reinforcing, more appealing. This, in turn, will contribute to the loosening and weakening of the old patterns and their hold on you.

But this process will not come without some difficulty and resistance. Change of any kind, even positive change, can be uncomfortable. To help you move forward in the face of this discomfort, I will address your fears as well as support you in your development of the courage to tolerate discomfort and let go of the old. The visualization process, in which you see and imagine the new brain growth, will further this development.

BEING IN THE MOMENT

At the heart of being on The Path is your ability to be in the moment. PGs are reinforced and maintained by our ongoing tendency to live life on automatic. We go through life doing things the same way day in and day out. We become entranced to go through each day the same way we did the day before. We love the familiar. We gravitate to what's comfortable, to what we know, to what we've done time and again. Living life in this manner will continually yield the same results you've gotten in the past and up until this point.

Right now, notice who is behind the eyes moving across this page—the "I" that is doing the reading, or listening to the audio book. Be aware of yourself right now in this moment. Focus on your breathing and watch your breath as you inhale and exhale. The part of you that, right now, is watching; the part that is observing yourself following my words. That's the part of you that we need to call on to begin living more in the moment. WAKE UP! This is what gives you the ability to make choices. And only by making choices can you begin to step out of the old patterns and step onto The Path.

When I was a kid in school I was fascinated by the concept of compounded interest. I remember a teacher holding up ten dollars and demonstrating how much you would have in ten years if that money compounds once a year. Then she recalculated, based on once a month compounding; then once a week, and once a day. In her last example, she compounded the interest once an hour. With each example, the same ten dollars, over the same period of time, turned into larger and larger amounts. When she compounded the money each hour, those ten dollars turned into millions. Wow, the more frequently you compounded, the greater the growth. I got it!

It's the same thing with awareness and presence. The more moments of your life you are present . . . the more frequently you WAKE UP to life : . . the greater the choice points for change and growth, and the greater the growth.

The Path is a process for enhancing awareness and empowering choices and having them compound moment by awakened moment. I will teach you a strategy of thinking that will help you deal with procrastination, worry, and everyday distractions. I hope to help you identify emotional unfinished business that causes you to overreact in social situations, while giving you the tools and step-by-step processes to help you resolve these emotional whirlpools. Ultimately, The Path is a process for the enhancement and directing of your brain's neuroplasticity, its ability to create new nerve cells and new nerve connections.

WHAT DO YOU WANT IN LIFE?

Whatever your goals, this book will help you get them, enjoy them, and keep making them better. Here are the nine things you will gain:

1. Pillar One: A better relationship with yourself
2. Pillar Two: Better relationships with others
3. Pillar Three: A more defined purpose in life and a stronger sense of interconnectedness
4. Pillar Four: A more efficient use of energy, improved sleep patterns, a greater ability to relax, and a greater ability to recover after stress
5. Pillar Five: A positive attitude and greater control over your thoughts
6. Pillar Six: Resolution of emotional issues and less reaction to life situations, resulting in less anxiety and depression
7. Pillar Seven: Ability to be more present in life and live in the moment
8. Pillar Eight: Greater flexibility to adapt to the ever-changing conditions of life
9. Pillar Nine: More "power," which I define as the ability to get things done

One of the hallmarks of primitive Gestalts and, indeed, of most childhood training and development is a focus on external judgments. We continually question ourselves based on what we think others are thinking. We continually judge ourselves in comparison to others. The consequence of this life strategy is that we don't give ourselves the opportunity to develop from the inside.

One of the keys to resilience, optimal living, and rejuvenation is the process of reaching inside and opening to the deepest parts of yourself.

This is the source of your creativity and even the birthing of new nerve cells. This is the source of your self-confidence and trust in the ability to let go, which further results in the optimal flow of energy throughout your body. One of your jobs along The Path is to begin "pruning back" the thicket of old thoughts and behaviors that slow your progress on The Path. This will lead you to true internal wisdom.

I would like to end this introductory chapter by congratulating you on your intention to grow and develop yourself in a healthy way. As you will learn in this book, the use of intention will facilitate the directing of gene expression—the actual manifestation of your genetic makeup. I would like to encourage you to keep this book next to your bed. Carry it with you and find time each day to read and refer to it. This book can change your life. I encourage you to give it that opportunity. You will be rewarded on many levels.

Right now, before you enter The Path, I'd like you to complete my Symptom Checklist and also my Resilience Questionnaire. They will be found in the appendix on page 373. This will mark your starting point in this process. You will be given opportunities to retake them later in the book so you can determine your progress on The Path.

After completing the Symptom Checklist, notice how many and which symptoms you have marked with a 3, 4, or 5. After completing my forty-item Resilience Questionnaire, total your scores for each of the 9 Pillars of Resilience in the boxes labeled "Total Score." Plot these scores on The Path of Resilience Profile that follows. It will give you a quick picture of the components of my model that are your strengths and which are areas needing development.

CHAPTER 2

"THE PATH" AND GUIDING YOU ONTO IT

I magine that your journey through life follows a path. You are on that path right now! Most of the time, however, this path is unplanned and unmarked. Typically, you are not aware of the path you are on. That's because your unconscious habit patterns "lead" you on an automatic path. As a result, you frequently find yourself where you don't want to be, which creates unnecessary stress, distraction, and wasted energy. And this is true even for the most successful of you.

I encounter those who believe that, because they have goals, they have created the path they are following. But this is belied by all the "successful" executives who approach me for counseling when their successes leave them short of happiness or suffering from sleepless nights, nagging physical symptoms, and unfulfilled relationships.

Your path is made up of successive moments in time that, placed end to end, comprise your journey through life. Now, you may ask if

I'm talking about your physical path, say, growing up in Cleveland and moving to Los Angeles. Or you might conceive of this as your career path through schools and into business or some profession.

While these are the concrete results you can point to in your life, I'm referring to a psychological concept, an emotional-mental-spiritual and physical state of being that you experience en route to the goals or destinations of your life. It is more of the "how" and the "why" than the "what" of your life. In fact, it reflects your quality of life and your effectiveness in it.

"The Path"—the one we are creating in this program—is described by a string of successive moments lived optimally. When I refer to "The Path," I'm referring to and defining your optimal functioning at any moment, based on the nine pillars' underlying resilience. This is The Path that results in a sense of joy, wholeness, optimal aging, and all dimensions of success.

Once you learn to identify The Path and the signposts that let you know if you are on or off it, you will feel a sense of reassurance. Those who don't have this path wander around. They suffer; they don't know where to go or how to make the best choices or decisions. When they take time off, they may feel uncomfortable, like they should be doing something more productive. By identifying what it takes to be on The Path, you have a "way." If you can adopt this path, it will give you faith, trust, and confidence in what you are doing. You will be very happy that you have a path. This is liberating. It can infuse you with a sense of power to know that you are going in the right direction and doing the right thing. This also removes considerable uncertainty in your life, your actions, and your decisions, further reassuring you and reducing your anxiety and worry. Your life will flow more smoothly. In addition, others will begin to feel this power and reassurance, this faith you have in yourself. A snowball effect will occur, in which your ability to be on The Path and your resultant confidence will be projected out and have a ripple effect. You will begin to note how others respond positively to you.

You can generate this sense of power every day of your life, every time you are present with The Path. In other words, your recognition that you chose The Path will lead you to this sense of power.

THE OPTIMAL PATH

When I refer to "The Path," I'm not referring to one path that everyone should take. The Path does not, in any way, suggest a specific way for you to live or lead your life. The Path, as I am referring to it, addresses how you are in the world and how you engage with the world. We can refer to this in a different way by identifying your contact boundary—in fact, two contact boundaries: the one where you and the outside world meet, and the one where you connect with your inner world. The optimal path, or being on The Path, means that you engage with your external and internal world with complete awareness and "response-ability." By "response-ability," I mean that you take responsibility for your life, and your presence is not impaired by past wounding or future worries. These cause a distraction that interferes with your ability to fully respond. Being on The Path means that you are fully able to notice and respond to any demand placed upon you. It also means you engage in the most appropriate management of your personal energy, or what I refer to as your "life force."

If I am defining "The Path" as the optimal route, then most of the time you are somewhere off this path and on another, going in a less than optimal direction—or simply wandering in the wilderness (metaphorically speaking). Let me give you some examples of what I'm referring to. If you have insecurities, you might awaken in the morning and worry about your day or a specific event, such as a meeting later in the day. This worry results in physical tension, nervousness, and the activation of your body's stress response.

It also distracts from your present moment—the only place where real living and joy take place. As I find with many of my clients, you may walk into your kitchen where family members want to be with you and talk with you. Instead, your preoccupations interfere with this contact, leaving your family feeling neglected and possibly rejected. Thus, you are off The Path (again, defined as the optimal way of being in the moment).

Another example is engaging in catastrophic thinking by imagining the worst possible outcome and focusing on it. This can lead to procrastination and avoidance. It not only creates fear, but it also triggers your body's stress response. It sends adrenaline through your body, tensing muscles, and raising heart rate and blood pressure. This creates unnecessary wear and tear on your body: You age more quickly and become fatigued way too fast. Thus, once again, you are off The Path. Now, you might be saying, "Wait a minute. I'm not a Pollyanna. Life can be dangerous, and I must always be prepared for what can happen, what can go wrong."

This point is well taken; life is full of uncertainty. We don't know exactly what to expect, and bad things can happen. It is important to anticipate and plan for future problems. Here the operative word is "plan." However, once you have done the appropriate planning, going over the plan again and again can be termed "worry" and obsessive thinking. I find that even when things are going well, our tendency is to worry about what might go wrong. We sacrifice enjoying success or happiness in the moment in order to "be prepared" for something that might go wrong in the future. Beyond planning, additional time and energy devoted to worry is counterproductive and takes you off The Path.

This point was continually demonstrated during the 2010 Winter Olympics in Vancouver. The athletes took risks every time they competed. In fact, in order to have any shot at a medal, athletes must go all out and completely clear their heads of the ongoing possibility of falling or making a mistake. When asked, one American Olympic athlete, Julia Mancuso, said, "You can't be scared!" In fact, this is what makes Mancuso and her peers truly Olympic athletes: that ability to put fear and danger out of their minds. The danger exists, but focusing on that danger serves no purpose and, in fact, impairs performance.

We can use these peak performers as exemplary models. The lesson is that optimal performance comes from being totally in the moment, despite the danger—not because the danger isn't real, but because focusing on the danger creates tension and ambivalence and has no constructive benefit. Thus, the other lesson is that optimal performance, or optimal functioning for the rest of us, begins with the ability to let go of everything but what's right in front of us. Learning this lesson will be addressed in the fifth pillar of resilience, mental balance and mastery, as well as in the seventh pillar, presence. These are all part of being on The Path.

THE IMPACT OF CHILDHOOD EXPERIENCE: PRIMITIVE GESTALTS

The path you are on is the result of what you learned during your early childhood experience; it is your reaction and conditioning to the rewards and punishments you received from others. Early on, it's mostly from your primary caregivers—mother and father. In other words, the path you take is determined by the rules laid down in your childhood environment. These are the rules most likely to maintain approval or avoid pain and punishment. They may be useful and important in your childhood environment, but they are not the best strategies for optimal living as an adult. In fact, much of the time, the path you take is an effort to avoid emotional pain and rejection while trying to win approval. This creates unnecessary physical, emotional, and mental strain that lowers your level of resilience. It also inhibits your behavior, causing you to shrink from new possibilities that make you uncomfortable. Some typical lessons learned in childhood include:

- The world isn't safe.
- It's not OK to be angry.
- Men shouldn't cry.
- Always be on guard.

- It's not OK to make mistakes.
- You are responsible for the feelings of others.
- Don't accept compliments because you may become too cocky.
- You are not OK; you are flawed.
- You can't get anything right.
- You are prone to making mistakes.
- You make bad decisions.
- You must be productive all the time.
- You will never be successful.
- You are not lovable.
- You don't deserve.

These early childhood lessons shape the development of your brain as well as your behavior. It is during this early stage of life that brain circuits, sometimes referred to as "cell assemblies," are reinforced (i.e., become associated with success: getting your needs met or avoiding punishment and pain). These cell assemblies gain strength, and those circuits and brain cells that are not reinforced disappear. In other words, your developing brain is a reflection of the world in which you grew up. Once established early in life, these patterns become more and more difficult to shift. After all, they were learned during your earliest survival efforts and are literally imprinted in your brain. Furthermore, the development of these patterns began before you were able to verbalize the lessons; thus, they sit in your body as feelings—making them even more difficult to recognize.

I refer to these patterns, which have a neuroanatomical foundation, as "primitive Gestalts." "Gestalt" is a German word that means "whole" or "complete." We can use the analogy of atoms. Atoms have protons in the center, which carry a positive charge, and electrons circling the center, which carry a negative charge. An atom requires an equal number of electrons and protons to be in balance. When an atom has fewer electrons than protons, it is unstable. We can say that it is in need of additional electrons. It will then have a tendency to combine with another atom, such that the combination produces a molecule in which there are an equal number of electrons and protons. In other words, there is an equal positive and negative charge that prevents both the loss or gain of additional electrons or protons. The molecule, we say, is in balance and thus resistant to further change.

Similarly, your primitive Gestalts "feel" complete, because they have given you needed survival answers and solutions. They feel right. That's because your observing self—your "I"—is embedded in the primitive Gestalt. When you go inside to check if something is right or not, you are comparing with the lessons and feelings of your childhood. (Remember, this is an unconscious process, so you probably don't even know you are doing it!) Thus, if the lesson was that getting close to another person is not safe (if you experienced abuse or even excessive criticism as a child), then as soon as you find yourself getting close in a relationship, it starts to feel uncomfortable. This discomfort leads to some action—such as finding something to argue about—that creates distance in the relationship. Even though this is destructive, it "feels right." You might even come up with a judgment about the actions of the other person to validate and reinforce the triggered feeling.

Let's look at an example. Take the case of Ed (not his real name), whose parents got divorced when he was nine years old, with the father leaving and having minimal contact after that. This loss was traumatic and painful. In an attempt to minimize the chances of suffering another loss of this magnitude—and the expectation that people close to him may leave—he made the decision never to get so close to another person that he or she could hurt him by leaving or rejecting him. (A similar decision can also come about because of an abusive or overly critical parent.)

There were two lifelong consequences of this decision. First, whenever Ed stayed in a relationship, he became more and more uncomfortable. His tendency was to cause conflict or do something to end the relationship before he got rejected. Second, he learned—unconsciously—not to notice this discomfort by numbing himself emotionally. One of the ways he did this was by developing a shallow and constricted breathing pattern. This resulted in him taking less oxygen into his body. By depriving every cell in his body of its normal supply of oxygen, he was partially deadening his body. This successfully created a numbing, which, throughout his life, he experienced as depression. Again, here we see a person living off The Path.

Primitive Gestalts "lock in" ways of thinking and behaving. In your early attempts at security and survival, they create answers to immediate needs. Fritz Perls, who helped found the Gestalt therapeutic approach, noted that as children we swallow messages (from parents and society) whole, without chewing or tasting. You make these "rules of living" your own, like the rules identified above. The conclusions you reach interfere with growth. As a result, primitive Gestalts and their neuroanatomical representations interfere with you getting your true needs met and achieving true completion. We might also say that they limit your ability to adapt or learn new lessons, a key to resilience.

Another client—let's call her Jane—demonstrates another common pattern. Jane's mother was very critical and unloving. She sometimes was angry with Jane for no apparent reason. No matter what this client did, there was no change in her mother's behavior. When she came home from school with a report card that was almost perfect, the mother complained about the single B on the card. Even all As did not achieve the love and connection Jane so desired. What were the consequences of this experience? Jane's first response was to try to anticipate her mother's every reaction and emotion. Through this process she became very sensitive to the slightest expressions of others and felt responsible for them. Second, she tried to get everything right so she wouldn't be criticized. When her behavior didn't get the response she wanted, no matter what she did, she simply tried to do more and do it better—of course, assuming that there was something wrong with her, not with her mother.

This pattern set the client off on an approach to life in which she always needed to be perfect and always be productive. Related to this is the type A person, who only feels as good as his or her last accomplishment. In both of these cases, an adult is still trying to receive the acceptance and approval that were elusive during childhood. The lack of such approval as a child left the adult with a sense of not being OK and not being deserving.

These paths and their consequences as described are incompatible with resiliency. We can therefore say these individuals are off The Path. In this program, I want you to begin identifying what would be The Path for you, to distinguish or discriminate when you are on The Path, versus the familiar path you have been on and are programmed to continue. Part of this process is to begin labeling aspects of your current path as being inappropriate—and the result of your primitive Gestalt pattern.

Even when you are successful, say in business, you may still be operating off The Path. I see many "successful" executives who are living unhappy, unfulfilled, stressful lives. The patterns developed early in life to survive and get by become fixed neurophysiological patterns. Think of a big field filled with thick bushes—except for the path that you keep taking. This path, because it is heavily traveled and heavily used, is beaten down and easy to walk on. So, even though you may feel unhappy or overwhelmed by life, and even though this path isn't taking you where you want to go, you continue to take it, because it's easy, familiar, comfortable, and automatic! And you aren't sure another way would be better—because there is no other clear path.

ASKING ONE QUESTION

Staying with this analogy, the direction that ultimately will lead to true success and happiness, because it is a new path, is typically a thicket that requires effort to make progress and get through to the other side. You are thus inclined not to take it because it is more difficult, unfamiliar or, more precisely, because it is unknown.

To help you through this thicket, we need to make it less formidable by giving you tools to cut the thicket, to make the unknown known, and to show you that it isn't as dangerous as you might imagine. Furthermore, I want to give you the hope and expectation that taking this new path will more likely lead you to your true goals in life and to true happiness. And finally, once you are on this path, you will discover that it actually makes your life much easier. This is sometimes referred to as being "in the flow." This will be illustrated shortly as you are asked to take the steps that put you onto The Path, where it will actually be easier to move forward in your life.

This optimal path I'm referring to is something that needs to be learned and cultivated. You will also need continual reminders because your natural tendency will be to fall back into the old habitual behaviors/path. In fact, we can say that your existing path, or pattern, has a gravitational pull. Even when you try to move away from it, it is always exerting strings of attachment. There is a name for this in scientific theory about how the world works. It's called an "attractor state," when an existing pattern has a strong pull, and you are continually attracted to and pulled back to it.

Success is often measured by the bottom line, a step up the corporate ladder, or more money in the bank. In my Resilience model of life and optimal living, however, those accomplishments represent only one aspect of success and of being on The Path. For example, in pillar three, you will learn that your relationship with "something greater" helps create a sense of wholeness and connection in your life. This is the opposite of the sense of isolation many of us feel, even with a big bank account.

Remember, this is not a program to help you become successful in business, make a lot of money, get the big house, or improve your image—even though following The Path will achieve all these goals as well. This is the resilient path—the path of optimal living. This path has broader values and goals that take into account physical health, emotional balance, relationships, and mental strength. The Path leads you away from a life in which you discard happiness in order to get ahead. No matter how much you need to get done, to resolve, finish, etc., it all starts with this very "moment," when you determine "Am I on The Path or off The Path?" And then you take the steps to get back on it, if you need to.

Thus, there will always be a simple discrimination that needs to be made. That is, whether you are in your old pattern, operating out of your primitive Gestalt—the automatic, habitual pattern of your existing path. Or whether you are consciously choosing new, healthy behaviors and a more positive, constructive path. Learning to discriminate between the two paths will coincide with the development of a new, healthier pattern, which I can assure you is underpinned by new brain development and my nine-component model of Resilience.

You are now ready to step onto The Path. On this path, which you will follow in practical steps throughout this chapter, you will begin taking more effective steps in your life and in your daily actions. At important points in the discussion, I will direct you onto The Path to address each step along the way, and then you will return to the explanations and continue.

PREPARING TO STEP ONTO THE PATH: YOUR FIRST TRUE STEP!

Here is your decision and your choice. Ask yourself these questions:

- Do I want to live in a more optimal fashion?
- Do I want to get unstuck?
- Do I want to handle stress more effectively and feel healthier?
- Do I want to reboot my ability to adapt and handle situations more effectively?
- Do I want to get my personal development process into high gear—be more aware, more awake, and more connected?
- Do I want to attract more positive results in my life?
- Do I want to have more satisfying relationships?
- Do I want to be more successful and resilient?
- Do I want to be happy and feel good about myself?

If you answered yes to these questions, here is the more difficult question to ask yourself: "Am I willing to expend time, effort, and attention in order to achieve these results?" If I give you a surefire path, will you commit to exerting effort in order to achieve these positive changes? Your effort is the price you pay for becoming resilient and achieving success, your life goals, and true happiness. (Keep in mind that when you are off The Path, you will be less efficient and less effective in life. So even though you may not realize it, you will waste much more energy with fewer positive results.)

If you are willing to make an effort, you are ready to continue with this book and The Path. Here you will complete step one: Declaring and solidifying your decision. Many years ago I went up to the frigid north to be an assistant professor at McGill University in Montreal. I had the good fortune to get there just before Donald Hebb retired and, even better, to get to know him. Hebb wrote one of the seminal books in the field of neuroscience, *The Organization of Behavior*. From this came his most paraphrased statement: "Neurons that fire together wire together." It is commonly referred to as "Hebb's law." This concept, which has been validated in many ways in recent years, illustrates the importance of making statements or thinking thoughts that we want to become reality. By making these statements, we create and then reinforce neuronal connections that they represent in the brain. That makes them more likely to occur in real life. This is what you are going to do in this first step on The Path.

STEP 1 *Declaring I want to be resilient and successful and to take the steps necessary for my greater development*

This first step is your creation of written "affirmations" to support your decision to live a more resilient and optimal life, and to make the necessary effort to achieve resilient success. Affirmations are statements that acknowledge beliefs you either hold to be true or want to believe are true. Affirmations are statements written "as if" they are already true. You then speak these messages to yourself on a regular basis.

As you constantly repeat these messages, your brain will lay down neural circuitry based on these statements. As a result, your brain will experience them as real and already taking place. They are a foregone conclusion. You are engaging in a dress rehearsal for optimal living.

Here are suggested affirmations for step one (use these or create similar statements that are a better fit for you). Write them on small index cards that you keep with you at all times. Meditate on them when you awaken, when you go to sleep, and at your three daily meals:

"I am living a more resilient and optimal life."

"I am making the necessary effort to be more resilient and function optimally."

"I am willing to make an effort and take actions to become resilient and successful."

STEP TWO: ADDRESSING YOUR SELF-SABOTAGE

Your success requires the full alignment of motivations, which can be expressed as a sense of deserving. As you will learn, you frequently carry around a part of yourself that is self-critical. We might even consider it self-destructive and undermining. This is the part that says "I am not good enough" or that continually reminds you of past mistakes. It is part of your primitive Gestalt. Consciously, you might say you are only trying to hold yourself accountable but, in fact, you are only holding yourself back.

Continually reminding yourself of past mistakes, thinking of yourself as bad, incompetent, or incapable, sends one message: "I don't deserve." Self-critical thoughts or comments are like digging the dirt out from under your foot after you work hard to take a step up the mountain. No matter how hard you work, these thoughts will interfere with forward progress. You must come from a place of "I deserve."

This step, therefore, helps with your ownership of "I deserve." This is important in order to eliminate any internal conflict and self-sabotage. Acknowledging that you deserve doesn't mean that you are perfect or without problems. Deserving is a natural right of everyone. The only thing it requires is intention and making a strong effort at personal improvement.

Right now, are you able to make the statement, "I deserve to be resilient and successful in my life"? Notice how you feel when you say this. If you feel any discomfort, resistance, or lack of conviction, it's important to explore what's causing this.

For many, this is a common stumbling block. It is due to messages of not being OK or of inadequacy that you are holding on to from your childhood. These messages are a constant companion through your own internalization process and development of your internal voice. Some of you are aware of these messages; for others, this is a new concept. But they are a factor in everyone's life. So let's take a moment right now to explore the messages you give yourself. Step two on The Path takes you through a process to uncover your hidden or not-so-hidden interference.

I take step two of the process from my work in Gestalt therapy. We use an empty chair to create a dialogue between two parts of yourself. Normally the voice of your primitive Gestalt is the only voice you hear. It has the power. It might be abusive, saying you don't deserve, or it might be subtle or even sneaky, saying, "Well, you would deserve if you didn't make so many mistakes," or "You would deserve if you worked a little harder." It can make itself very "reasonable" but in truth, the message is: you don't deserve.

This voice of your primitive Gestalt will sit in one chair. In the other is your healthy voice heard less often. When you stay in the familiar voice, it masks or drowns out the other. Your familiar voice represents and supports the old pattern. By creating this dialogue, you get to hear the new voice that you want to support and strengthen—the voice that truly wants good things for you. Go to step two to be guided through this process.

STEP 2 *Addressing self-sabotage*

I'd like you to engage in a dialogue with yourself. It might help to actually shift chairs, placing the two parts of yourself in different chairs.

Let's identify these two parts. One is your healthy part, which bought this book and wants to become more resilient and successful. The second part of yourself can be critical, punitive, and even abusive at times. This is the part that uses more negative than positive adjectives to describe you. Or it will quickly add a "but" after any praise.

"Yes, but anyone could have done it," "Yes, but I was lucky." It is the part of yourself that may not feel that you are OK. In fact, it might still be blaming you for childhood mistakes and thinking that you are defective.

Now, start off by giving the positive part of you a voice and say, "I deserve to be resilient, successful, and happy." Notice how you feel as you say this. Next, shift to the other chair.

Become the part that can be critical and give this part a voice. This part might find something about you that is not OK: "You don't try hard enough; you aren't organized enough; you aren't nice enough; you're not focused enough; you're too lazy."

Continue with this dialogue by moving into the chair of the positive voice. Respond from this perspective and then continue switching back and forth. Notice any tendency to undermine your feelings of deserving. Notice, also, any feelings coming up toward the undermining voice. Finally, see if you can find new strength when speaking from the place of the positive voice.

We will return to this dialogue process and take it further in chapter seven when we address your relationship to yourself.

At this point, it is important simply to be aware that these two parts of you exist. Also, at this point, we need to be able to stand on the side of "I deserve to be resilient and successful" despite our ambivalence.

STEP THREE: "I DESERVE"

To facilitate the belief that you deserve, there must be the concept of acceptance. In this context, acceptance is the opposite of denial. We are in denial much of the time. Every time we are upset with ourselves for making a mistake, we are in denial. Every time you tell yourself you should be better than you are, you're coming from a place of denial. Let me explain.

The laws of physics (except in quantum physics, which we'll discuss later) say that you can be in only one place at a time. Typically you get upset at where you are on your developmental path, your life's journey. Every time you say, "I should have done better," you are saying you should be further along in your development. You "should" be better. This is denial. It is denying where you actually are on your path and saying that you should be further along. Acceptance is simply agreeing with and living by the basic principle that you can only be in one place at a time. If right now you typically misplace items such as your keys, then, right now, you are a person who does not pay attention and is absent-minded.

STEP FOUR: ACCEPTING YOUR PRESENT CIRCUMSTANCES IS ONLY ACCEPTING REALITY

In fact, every time you get angry with yourself for not performing better than you do, you undermine your growth. You are telling yourself that you are not OK, not good enough. This hurts your self-credibility and makes you less sure of yourself, making it more difficult for you to try new behaviors.

I'm not suggesting that acceptance means being satisfied with where you are or that you are not going to get better or do better. It's simply an acknowledgment of fact: "This is where I am right now, at this moment, with all my flaws. I do want to continue to grow and get better, but here is where I currently am." So, if you keep making mistakes or keep losing or misplacing things, that is who you are right at this moment: someone who has difficulty paying attention and being present.

By coming from a place of acceptance, you are being most supportive of yourself. You are better able to consciously look at yourself. (When we don't like who we are, we have greater difficulty seeing ourselves.) In fact, this is the shortest path for your optimal growth and achieving all that you want to accomplish.

Step four is the process of accepting yourself with all your warts. "Right now, this is who I am. I want to achieve greater awareness, make fewer mistakes, and generally function more optimally, but this is where I am right now." Another reason it's important to be accepting of yourself and your circumstances is that it helps you avoid getting overwhelmed by all of the problems you face or the massive changes you feel you need to make in order to be OK or successful.

So many of the people I work with will start out being discouraged by all the changes they feel they have to achieve before they can experience relief—or simply acceptance. The sense is that you're in a hole—perhaps you even feel you have dug this hole yourself. This perspective has you putting life on hold until you get out of the hole. Accepting where you are is a helpful breather for the moment in time and place. It gives you the ability to gain a sense of progress even early in this process. Go to The Path and take steps three and four now.

STEP 3   *I deserve this success.*

Suggested affirmations to write and repeat to yourself:

"I deserve to live a healthy and successful life."

"I deserve to feel good."

"I deserve to live without worry or tension."

STEP 4   *I am accepting of myself.*

Create affirmations or self-statements that support acceptance of yourself and where you are in your life. Here are some examples:

"Although it is difficult to look at myself and see myself with all my faults, I accept that this is where I'm at as I begin The Path."

"By accepting myself, I am taking the shortest route (The Path) to resilience and success."

"Although I make mistakes and am far from perfect, I completely and truly accept myself."

"Self-acceptance places me on The Path."

STEP FIVE: STEPPING ONTO THE PATH—INTENTION, YOUR FIFTH STEP

Here is where you bring in your intention, the part of you that wants something better, the part of you that wants a healthier, happier, and more successful life. This is an important step for many reasons. First, as noted previously, there are parts of you that unconsciously interfere with your forward progress. You may be aware of your self-sabotage, or you may have been blaming others or bad luck for being stuck. You have already taken the first step in a dialogue with the part of you that undermines. Intention is the countervailing force opposing the attractor state of the primitive Gestalt, your old pattern. It helps mobilize your power, your strength to be on The Path.

Let me make an even stronger statement about intentions. In quantum physics there is the concept of a quantum leap. An electron, for example, can "jump" from one atomic orbit to the next without moving through the intermediate space between electron orbits. One moment it's in one orbit, and in the next it's in another orbit. It's a matter of physics. We say the process is discontinuous. On the human subjective level, I believe it is intention that fuels your creative and developmental leaps. Furthermore, it is the active ingredient in loosening the hold your primitive Gestalt has on you.

Here is another way of thinking about intentions. Your unconscious mind responds to the intentions of your conscious mind. When you have a clear intention and follow a practice step-by-step, your conscious intention attracts the unconscious resources needed to change the state of your consciousness. Over time, the unconscious is impressed by conscious repetition.

Right now, let's focus on your intention! Having an intention is having a driving purpose in your mind. This directs your mind, giving it an aim and a powerful force. By setting your intention, you align the forces of the universe to help ensure your success in following The Path. Go to step five right now and write these new affirmations. Share your intentions with one person who is close to you.

STEP 5 | *Declaring my intention*

Self-statement: "I am declaring to myself and to others my intention to do whatever is necessary to make the effort, to get onto and stay on The Path—the optimal way for me to live my life and be resilient."

"I will devote myself to greater awareness and living from a place of intention and purpose."

"I will root out my thinking and behaviors that are not supportive of my highest intentions."

"I will share my purpose with at least one close relationship in order to make this declaration public and also to receive support in getting on and staying on The Path."

STEP SIX: REMEMBERING

Being on The Path requires continually choosing. But most of the time you are acting out of habit and unaware. Being on automatic results in following your old path and being unable to choose.

As I mentioned, your old pattern, your primitive Gestalt, has a gravitational pull. This means, plain and simple, that initially it has control. It is the default position. Without a consistent plan to remember to be on

The Path, you will automatically revert to the primitive Gestalt path. If the field you are going through is a jungle with thickets all around except for this one path, unless you make a conscious choice, your feet will do the walking—down the existing and easy path. You're in your old world!

So the challenge is remembering. Gurdjieff, an early twentieth-century mystic, referred to "remembering oneself." This is where you are able to see what there is to see, while noticing that you are seeing. It is a state of being self-aware and being a witness to yourself. Ordinarily, when you are engaged in life, you lose your sense of "I."

For this reason, the next step is remembering to notice whether you are on or off The Path—in other words, awaken to the moment for as many moments in your day as possible. Ideally, this can occur during important choice points. On a deeper level, this is a process of recognizing that you have choices in life. Typically it is a choice between your old, habitual behaviors and newer, intentional ones.

In these moments of choice, of "remembering" to notice, you can begin to observe how you are moving through your life. "On The Path" is the new pattern and "off The Path" is the old. For example, the old pattern may be to say no to doing something because it would be uncomfortable or scary—in short, out of your comfort zone. But this old pattern keeps you stuck and unsatisfied. Instead, decide to say yes!

Throughout the book, methods will be identified for you to remember to notice if you are on or off The Path. Part of this process will be to remember to take supportive actions that help you move forward on The Path. Right now, go to step six and take action.

STEP 6 *Creating a structure for remembering*

Until you develop greater self-awareness, you will need to create a structure for remembering. This will take the form of a series of three-by-five index cards on which you place your responses to the first steps: your affirmations, your self-statements, and your intentions.

Place these cards next to your bed so you will see them, read them, and meditate on them when you awaken in the morning.

Carry them with you during your day.

Take them out and read them at breakfast and lunchtime.

Take them out and read them at 3 PM.

Take them out and read them at dinnertime.

And finally, as you place them next to your bed when you go to sleep, read them a final time. By reading these statements right before going to bed, you are taking them to sleep with you and helping them enter your unconscious mind.

STEP SEVEN: ASK YOURSELF THE QUESTION

Am I on The Path? This is your ongoing question that establishes each moment as a moment for optimal functioning. A positive answer to this question will help you address any feelings of overwhelm in your life. Right now, you may be saying to yourself, "There is so much I need to accomplish in order to be resilient. I have to be more aware, I have to be more focused, I have to make fewer mistakes, I have to be more punctual . . ." and on and on.

If you approach each moment of your life with multiple demands and multiple expectations—if you sit down to do one task with a head filled with all the other things you need to do in life—these distractions will only create more tension and less effectiveness.

Resilience and peak performance begin with establishing a way to be completely present and satisfied, each and every moment of your life. This is the lesson behind The Path. No matter where you are in your development, in your progress, if you live this moment optimally you are considered to be on The Path. And that is the best that you can do, and it needs to be appreciated. Go to step seven to complete this chapter.

STEP 7 *Asking yourself the question*

The beauty of this program and being on The Path is that no matter where you are in your personal development, you can be successful. Even if you are having difficulty managing your life, you can still follow these steps and feel good about your efforts. This is because The Path is defined as being in the moment in the most optimal manner.

For example, right now, the most optimal manner is simply following the first six steps of this chapter.

So, how do you know if you are doing well enough? If you have taken the first six steps as outlined above, you are definitely on The Path!

So ask yourself:

"Am I on The Path?"

You have the power and the ability to make this true. Just follow the first six steps above—and then, move forward to the next chapter and the next steps, assured that you will be taking the shortest route toward resilience and optimal living.

"THE PATH" CHAPTER BY CHAPTER

Being on The Path means developing a healthy, resilient way of being in the world and supporting your progress toward life goals. In this chapter I've introduced you to your primitive Gestalt: your internal guide developed during childhood. It is represented by the voice you continually hear in your head, even when you don't notice it. This voice—the result of childhood training and survival learning—is typically inaccurate and inappropriate in your life as an adult. At the very least, it's like throwing an anchor behind you on your journey through life. Its presence, 24/7, is primarily responsible for maintaining old behavioral, mental, and emotional habits. It locks you into old messages you have about yourself. One of the goals of The Path is to recognize its inaccuracies and shift you away from your old internal guide to a healthier, more mature internal guide, which is a voice that develops as you go further down The Path, when a deeper knowing, awareness, or learning will occur. In fact, the use of intentions used in this book are designed to help you create a new vision and story about yourself.

The Path accomplishes two more important goals.

1. With each step you take on The Path, you will be learning to trust yourself. Thus, another benefit of The Path is the fostering of self-confidence. This occurs automatically when you do the right thing and then acknowledge to yourself that you did so. In other words, you are learning that you can rely on yourself. This is at the heart of self-confidence, one more step in the achievement of optimal living.

2. The other goal you will achieve is improved awareness and consciousness. As you learn to focus and be more confident, you will have less reason to escape and thus be more capable of being in the present moment, where all life takes place.

SIGNPOSTS

At the end of each chapter you will find "signposts." Just like road markers, they let you know that you are truly on The Path. They are clear demonstrations to yourself that you can do it, that you are doing it. They are your signposts for being on The Path.

SIGNPOST

- You have declared your desire to be resilient and successful.
- You have held a dialogue between the two parts of yourself.
- You have written an affirmation that you deserve to achieve success in this program.
- You have created a self-statement that supports acceptance of yourself.
- You have created an intention to do whatever is necessary to get onto and stay on The Path.
- You have created three-by-five cards to remember to engage in this program.
- You have asked yourself the question "Am I on The Path or off The Path?"

CHAPTER 3

THE CHALLENGE OF RESILIENCE AND OPTIMAL PERFORMANCE IN TODAY'S WORLD

No one needs to tell you that life is challenging and stressful. Or that the challenges of life take a toll on your body and your spirit. You might never have learned how to deal with stress during your years of schooling, but you certainly know how it feels. It might be a nagging muscle ache or just a tight muscle. It could show up as a worry, a distraction, or butterflies in your stomach. It may manifest in addictive or avoidance behaviors and a loss of motivation. You know when the stresses of life are keeping you up at night or distracting you from being in the present.

You know when you are experiencing more stress than you would like, or when you feel like the stress you're experiencing is more than you can handle. It can be overwhelming and draining. But either you haven't made the effort to gain control over these stresses, or your efforts have been less than fruitful.

Whether consciously or unconsciously, it's easy to throw up your hands in frustration, saying, "Life is simply stressful." More often than not, that sense of overwhelm prevents you from taking action. Even if you disregard the physical and emotional consequences, stress takes a toll on your performance.

In the next few pages I'll map out the territory of life's stresses to demonstrate their prevalence and magnitude; illustrate their impact on your health and your performance; and begin the process of learning awareness, seeing the possibilities, and attaining resilience. These are the first steps to riding the waves of life's challenges instead of wiping out in those waves.

ARE TODAY'S STRESSES WORSE THAN THOSE OF OUR "CAVEMEN" ANCESTORS?

Is this a fair question to ask? Many times I hear people talk about how the stresses of modern life are so much more intense than in the "old days." And I wonder if this is really a fair comparison. It's like the person living in a small, modern American home saying he doesn't have enough room. This would be laughable to someone living in a one-room hut in Haiti or Africa.

Yes, the stresses of modern life are incomparable when we look at their complexity. However, if we consider the most fundamental aspect of stress—the danger to survival—there is no comparison. As you move further back in time, true dangers to personal survival are ever more present.

For the caveman, survival was a daily struggle. Moment by moment, vigilance and concern for personal safety were an ongoing reality. Living in that most primitive environment, you could be attacked at any time by a predatory animal or someone challenging you for possession of your territory. Basic sustenance was a daily concern.

With no refrigerator or agriculture, it was difficult to save for a "rainy day" or the inevitable drought. With the arrival of an agricultural society, we begin to see a little bit of a buffer. If there was a good crop, you had a little bit of breathing room. But dangers to survival were still ongoing and uncertainty abounded.

Today, most of us don't struggle for personal survival on a daily basis. In fact, unlike our counterparts from the past, the odds are that we will survive to reach reproductive age. And for this development and degree of safety we must be grateful. We must be grateful and appreciative to live in relative freedom from immediate danger. It is our advantage. Thus, the first step on The Path for this chapter is an appreciation that few of our stresses are life-threatening, and that most of us have the basic necessities of life.

But that makes the stakes higher, in a sense. We don't simply want to live to see another sunrise or to reach reproductive age. We want to live much longer and healthier, into our eighties and beyond! In the "old" days, we might die of other causes before the impact of stress took its toll. Now, we have many more years for the destructive consequences of stress to develop. Also, today we experience a broader array of demands. And while they may not be life-threatening, we experience many of them with the same sense of urgency and fear.

STEP 1 *Having gratitude that your stresses are not life-threatening (with a caveat*)*

Whatever your stresses, you are not in danger of starving to death, being eaten by a tiger, or being threatened by someone trying to take over your territory (although sometimes in business it may feel that way).

Many of you experienced dangerous childhoods filled with uncertainty, crises, and perhaps even abuse. As a child, you were helpless to make the situation different.

But as we become adults, two things change: We have more ability and resources, and we can choose environments that have greater safety. In other words, there are fewer threats to our survival.

It's important, therefore, to acknowledge and appreciate this relative level of safety. And for this, I suggest a sense of gratitude. The more you tell yourself that you are safe, the more opportunity you give your body to breathe a sigh of relief and to feel good.

> *Caveat: The exception is if you or someone close to you has a life-threatening illness or perhaps an ongoing symptom or chronic pain. Yet, even in these situations, after you do whatever you can for your health, it is even more important to then "let go" and accept. Acceptance frees your body to devote all of its energy to the healing process.*

TODAY'S BACKGROUND STRESSES

Stress presents itself in many ways and on many levels. Some levels we are completely unaware of. Psychology presents us with a classic study of what happens when you add more rats to a cage. As the number of animals increases, there is a predictable increase in aggression and mortality. Crowdedness, as this demonstrates, is a source of stress. We can observe this as the number of cars on the road increases, or as we walk in a crowd or make our way through a crowded room.

Crowdedness, or the increase in population density, is only one aspect of the growing complexity and pressures we face in the world today. We notice it in the speed of communication—which requires a more rapid response—and we notice it in the amount of information we encounter on a daily basis. This gives us the feeling that there is always something we need to do. This is stressful!

With increasing complexity, it takes longer for us to complete tasks. We are therefore left with a growing list of unfinished business. Each item on this list requires some attention and serves as yet another distraction from being present and in the moment—and creates another source of worry: "Can I actually meet the demands placed on me?"

External factors also include the ongoing stream of bad news we are faced with through TV, radio, newspapers, and the ever-expanding information threads of the internet. Suddenly we have become witness to bombings halfway around the world. When a war breaks out in Europe or the Middle East, or an earthquake and tsunami occur in Japan, we see the tragedy unfolding in real time. It is impossible to view images of suffering without it having an impact on our emotions, even if we quickly bury these feelings.

We see death, the ultimate source of stress, on a daily basis. (While car crash fatalities of strangers may not cause us to grieve, they do remind us that when we get into our cars there is a chance that we will get killed. That's especially true if the report in the media is about someone who ran a red light or who was driving under the influence, because these are situations out of our control.) This is the backdrop of uncertainty and danger that is an ongoing reality in our lives. Before you even begin to address your specific life stresses, notice (step two) how they sit on top of the stresses of modern life.

STEP 2 *Noticing what impacts you*

Unless you are living somewhere in the woods far from a city, you are affected by aspects of our advanced civilization that can be stressful. These include excessive noise, traffic, crowdedness, violence, and crime, along with all the bad news we hear about through various avenues of communication.

As a way of acknowledging the diversity of the stimuli that impact you and can create tension and distraction, let's take a little tour of your own "noticing." Do you have to deal with environmental challenges? Noise? Crowding? Air or other pollution? Crime and safety concerns? Do you have traffic or transportation stress? Are you aware of civic strains—conflicts in your community?

Do you feel impacted by government corruption or stagnation—an inability to solve problems? Does awareness of the houseless or the mentally ill in your community disturb you? How does the constant stream of hardships you hear about from around the world affect you? Do you experience some emotional upset when you hear about the tragedies of others? As I have already mentioned, it's impossible not to be affected. Take a moment to allow yourself to be present with any emotions that come up during this assessment.

WHAT IS STRESS ANYWAY?

There are many misconceptions about stress. With all the publicity on the subject, one can easily get the message that stress is bad and should be eliminated. At the same time, we seem to look for and even desire stress. How is it possible to reconcile these two positions? The quick and dirty answer is that stress is a necessary and even helpful part of life. In fact, it's almost impossible to achieve success without encountering a certain amount of stress. It prepares you for danger, but, more important, it mobilizes your body for action. It helps sharpen your senses to take in more information and be more vigilant. And, within limits, it improves performance. The problem occurs when you lose control over your stresses, when you place too much stress on yourself, and when you don't allow your body to recover appropriately from these stresses. Problems also occur when you maintain defensive patterns based on childhood learning and don't adjust to the new realities of your adult life.

Let me present a brief definition of stress so you can see why it has become such a buzzword in our language and an influence on our lives. Anything that is a potential source of danger is a source of stress, referred to as a "stressor," or "stress trigger" (in other words, it's something that triggers your stress response).

To protect yourself from this danger, your body prepares to either fight the danger or flee from it. Your body's response can be considered your stress reaction, or stress response, to these demands. Your stress response can be triggered by an automobile cutting in front of you, a deadline at work, conflict in a relationship, or a death in the family.

Stress is also caused by positive events, such as getting a promotion, taking on a challenging or exciting project, getting married, and having a baby. Yes, stress can occur as a result of both good events and bad events—after all, if you get promoted at work there is typically an escalation in demand and expectation, which can be experienced as danger, particularly if you are concerned about your ability to meet that demand. Hans Selye, the person who coined the word "stress" for human behavior, made the distinction between good and bad stress, calling one's response to something good "eustress."

YOUR STRESS RESPONSE

Let's talk about your stress response, which is a biological and necessary mechanism for survival. In the broadest sense of the word, stress results from any demand to adapt, change, and mobilize either physically or emotionally for danger and threat. Your stress response prepares you to overcome the danger. This response was first described by Walter Cannon over a hundred years ago as the "fight-or-flight response" because, as mentioned, it prepares the body to either fight or run from the danger.

Here are things you might notice when you're stressed: When you avoid another car while driving, notice the speeding up of your heart and the tight grip of your hands on the steering wheel. If you are meeting a date for the first time, you might notice the same response. Notice whether your hands get moist or clammy. If your boss just reprimanded you, you might notice sweating under the collar or a kink in your neck.

If you are in your car and are late for an appointment, or just worried about the appointment, you might notice tension in your jaw. If you have a meeting tomorrow in which a lot of money is dependent upon a good performance, you might become tense and engage in thoughts called "worry"—which might make it difficult for you to fall asleep. Take some time to go onto The Path and do steps three, four, and five.

STEP 3 *How easily does your stress response get triggered?*

Awareness is the first step in making any changes in your behavior. Awareness makes the unconscious conscious. This is a prerequisite to responding differently or thinking differently. After all, you must notice an inappropriate thought or action before you can make any adjustment.

Pay attention to your stressors, or stress triggers, today. But do it from the position of an objective witness.

What triggers your stress response at work? Is it a concern about the judgments of others? When you are meeting people, do you get nervous or tense? Do you jump to what can go wrong, rather than what can go right?

Think about your day. How easily do you get stressed, worried, or tense?

Notice your behavior without judgment. In fact, have a bit of compassion for what you go through.

STEP 4 *Your stress response*

Begin to pay attention to your body's particular response pattern to stress and preparation for danger. What do you notice when you are stressed, worried, or fearful?

Do you notice heart palpitations, sweaty hands, tense jaw or neck? Perhaps you are more easily distracted when stressed?

When you have a moment, go to the Symptom Checklist you completed after chapter one. Notice which signs of stress you are exhibiting.

STEP 5 *The mismatch*

What was the last stressful experience you had in which it served you to prepare for fight or flight? When was your last opportunity to beat up someone to solve a problem? When were you able to address a stressful situation by running away from it?

Notice the mismatch between how your body is wired to respond to stress (the legacy from our hunter/gatherer ancestors) and what is typically required to deal with your stresses. There is typically a much bigger response than is needed. Most of your stresses are best handled by a calm focus and awareness.

As you can see, a stressful event can trigger a host of reactions long before the actual event. We have a tendency to activate to a stress, even if that stress is far in the future. All it takes is thinking about it, and your body wants—no, it insists—on mobilizing.

When you complete a business meeting or a school presentation, but the results are not immediately determined; if you review the experience and are critical of your performance; if you focus on your mistakes; or if you begin to anticipate a negative response, you will maintain the stress long after the performance. This is because your body is still preparing for danger. Your biological survival mechanism gets triggered and prolonged by any potential danger. This is in contrast to the resilient person, whose body shifts into recovery after the stress is over. Your body can either be in protective mode, or heal, grow, and recover.

Let's take a closer look at what happens inside your body when it gears up for danger:

When your brain detects or determines that there is a threat, it sends a message to the pituitary gland deep within your brain. Here is where ACTH (adrenocorticotropic hormone) is produced and released into the bloodstream, where it arrives at the adrenal glands. Here, adrenaline and other hormones are released to help prepare you for the expected demands. For example, your heart rate and blood pressure increase to allow more blood to flow to muscles that are expected to be used to handle the threat or demand placed on your body.

Sugars and fats are released into the blood to deliver nutrients to the muscles, which tense up in preparation for confronting the threat. This process is facilitated by an increase in breathing rate to supply more oxygen to these muscles. Finally, your nervous system goes on the alert, and your eyes dilate to take in more information and be able to react more quickly to the threat.

As part of this process, your cardiovascular system (heart and blood vessels), the neuromuscular system (muscles and the nerves that direct them), and autonomic nervous system (control center of the body) step into action. At the same time, systems in your body not necessary for immediate protection will shut down. These include your digestive system and your reproductive system. It's circle-the-wagon time, with very little energy available for growth.

And even though food and digestion are needed for long-term survival, you are not thinking of your dinner when you're trying to avoid being lunch for a tiger. You might also notice that your immune system doesn't seem to work well when you are stressed—leading to you getting more colds or the flu.

It is interesting to note that one enzyme released into the blood speeds up the rate at which the blood will clot. Now, here is a perfect example of the different needs of present-day stress versus the stress experienced by our ancestors. This increase in the ability of the blood to clot is clearly useful and even lifesaving if the danger results in attack and you are injured. This enzyme will help the blood clot faster, thus reducing the chances you will lose too much blood.

This same adaptive ability for your blood to clot, however, can be dangerous for hypertensive patients, whose doctors try to thin their blood so it can pass more easily through narrowed arteries.

As you can see, these changes require energy. So, the body must work extra hard to produce this stress response. It uses the body's adaptation energy or "survival energy" to accomplish this. Earlier, I used the term "life force" to refer to this energy.

In fact, about 1,400 biochemical changes take place in your body every time you initiate a stress response. So, while your body is adapted to support the stress response, it also requires recuperation from the effort and the effects of its activation. The solid line in Figure 1 (on page 49) shows the healthy pattern of activating to handle a stress and then deactivating to recover and restore resources used up during the stress response. When this happens in an appropriate way, the body is fully available when another stress demand occurs. When engaged in this pattern, the body doesn't suffer from the effects of stress. This is resilience at work.

Preparing for stress is important. Your body wants to adapt. It is the most important thing it does, along with reproduction. This is what allows you to survive long enough to reproduce. So your body has been developed to employ an excellent stress response. This involves all the things that help you cope and stay alive. In that case, what's the problem?

Well, just as you know that budgets need to be balanced, that there isn't an unlimited supply of money for you or even your government, you don't have an unlimited amount of adaptation energy. Many of you already know this because your level of energy does not seem to match your needs. Or you're too tense at night to fall asleep easily.

You see, after the threat that first triggers your stress response is over, your body needs to recuperate. This is a key component of resilience. Normal levels of muscle tension, heart rate, and blood pressure need to be restored.

Let's look again at Figure 1 on page 49, which also presents a pattern of behavior that is more familiar to you and most people you know, represented by a dashed line. Here, we handle stress, and then we are immediately faced with, or look for, another danger. And so, before any recuperation can take place, our stress response gets trig-gered again. At the end of this stress, the same thing happens: we immediately identify another demand, pressure, or danger that further triggers our stress response.

Notice that it doesn't matter how successful you are in dealing with each of these stresses (although failure presents us with a totally different array of difficulties). You quickly find yourself stretching the resources of your body. At this point, you are in danger of physiological burnout and damage. It also contributes to inflammation on a cellular level, the precursor to many illnesses.

Think of a rubber band. In fact, imagine right now holding a rub-ber band by your two thumbs. A rubber band is meant to stretch; this is its function, just as your body is meant to produce a stress response. But what happens to a rubber band after it is stretched? That's right; it needs to be released so it can return to its resting position. In this position, it's prepared to be used again.

Now imagine stretching the rubber band, pulling your thumbs farther away from each other and watching the rubber band stretch. Before releasing it, stretch it again . . . and again . . . and again. If you keep stretching the rubber band without allowing it to relax and return to its original position, what happens? With the rubber band stretched so taut, it is no longer flexible, no longer functional. At some point you will begin to see tears occurring and, ultimately, it will break.

Like the rubber band, your body must relax and recuperate after each stressful experience. When this process of balancing does not occur, three things tend to happen. First, like the overstretched rubber band, you stretch the resources of your body, and breakdown begins to occur. Your body's weakest genetic link will be the first system to show signs and symptoms of stress overload. A second thing that happens is a growing inability of your body to deeply relax. You are less and less able to feel a sense of calm. In fact, even when asleep many of us hold a certain level of tension. This creates an overall sense of dis-ease, lack of energy, and poor performance and motivation.

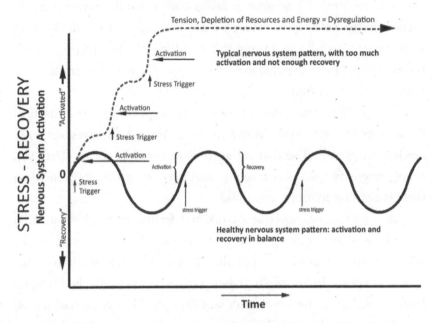

FIGURE 1 | Healthy stress with activation and recovery periods, and common harmful stress activation pattern with little or no recovery

Perhaps most important, changes take place in your brain that leave you more susceptible to new problems. As will be discussed in later chapters, the hippocampus is a special area of the brain where, among other functions, neurogenesis takes place.

Neurogenesis is at the heart of resilience and your brain's ability to learn, grow, and renew itself. Neurogenesis is nothing less than the birthing and developing of new nerve cells, the basic building blocks of your brain. Stress has been shown to impair the hippocampus's ability to produce viable new nerve cells.

The longer you go before your body has the opportunity to recover and for the different systems to rest, the greater the wear and tear on your body. Selye, who performed hundreds of scientific experiments related to stress, showed the breakdown of body organs following prolonged exposure to stress.

Herein lies the problem. We no longer give our bodies the opportunity to recover. We no sooner finish one stressful activity than we encounter the next. Even when we are not engaged physically with something stressful, we are probably thinking of something stressful. It is important to realize that even these thoughts will trigger the stress response just described: no rest for the weary!

Your problem intensifies as your body keeps trying to rid itself of the source of the stress you are dealing with. You see, the stress response mechanism is geared so that if the stress or threat is not resolved, you simply intensify the stress response and keep it on longer, even when there is nothing more for you to do.

Jason was an employee at a bank and feeling particularly stressed out. He was just making ends meet financially. At the end of the month, when it was time to pay the mortgage, he frequently had difficulty scraping the money together. His concerns intensified when a friend working at the same bank was laid off. He felt he had no job security and that he could be next.

Although Jason could not do anything about his current job, the possibility of being laid off and not having enough money to live on was a constant stress trigger. The key word here is "constant." He was not able to let go of his fears and thus was not able to turn off the stress response. So, even though the mobilization of his body did not increase his job safety, he was not able to turn it off.

Another example is the inappropriate muscle bracing that occurs when you are angry or frustrated. It uses up energy and causes the breakdown of tissue and cells without any positive benefits. This translates into the depletion of adaptation energy, with nothing to show for it. Do steps six through nine now.

STEP 6   *Assessing your level of adaptation energy*

Signals that indicate less than optimal levels include: poor sleep pattern (either delay in falling asleep or awakening before a full night's sleep), muscle tension or aches, fatigue or not enough energy to meet your needs, frustrations, worries, and distractions.

Take a moment to estimate and give yourself a score from 0 to 100, where 100 is optimal levels of adaptation energy and 0 is none.

STEP 7 *Your pattern*

How much do you scan your environment and your life to look for danger? Do you give yourself a break, particularly after completing a task? Or do you immediately go to the next problem, not allowing your body to take a breather?

STEP 8 *Stress triggers*

Review your last few days and identify situations that were stressful. Which people interactions caused tension? Which future events are worrying you?

STEP 9 *When do you relax?*

In the last few days, when did you find time to relax, to completely let go? This doesn't mean watching an action program on TV, but a time for focused relaxation.

IS STRESS GOOD OR BAD?

The answer is yes. Stress can be good and stress can be bad. The question should be: "What makes stress either good or bad?" Remember, the stress response is an adaptive response. It's one of the most important mechanisms in your body. For such an important adaptive response to develop through the evolutionary process, it must have special characteristics that enhance your performance.

Within limits, the stress response enhances your ability to take in information. It helps make you more alert and more focused. It strengthens your motivation and drive for success.

All people who are successful experience stress. That's because success always involves taking risks, which involve some danger and thus will trigger the stress response. To live life to the fullest, you cannot avoid all stressful situations. In fact, studies have found that people achieve peak performance when they are under a certain amount of stress. So you can see that you need stress in your life and that stress actually enhances it.

Here is where you begin to run into difficulty. In my search to understand my clients' tendencies to seek stress, I came across an important finding. Learning is a basic mechanism of life. When you figure something out, it is important to remember the lessons of the experience so that you don't have to keep relearning the same thing.

One type of learning is referred to as "classical conditioning." Most of you are familiar with the famous Russian scientist Igor Ivanovich Pavlov, who loved dogs and played with them a lot.

He also liked bells. So he decided to combine these two things that he loved: dogs and bells. In his now-famous experiment, every time he gave his dogs food, he rang a bell. So they heard the bell, and then their master, Pavlov, gave them food.

When we eat, we create saliva in our mouths to mix with the food and begin the digestive process. Dogs also salivate when they are eating. Pavlov decided to measure this saliva. After he rang the bell a number of times just before the dogs got their food, he then rang the bell without presenting their food (which wasn't very nice of him). What he found was that the dogs still salivated simply at the sound of the bell.

In other words, the bell became associated with the presentation of the food. And the dogs learned to associate the sound of the bell with the expectation of food: classical conditioning!

What does this have to do with stress and success? As I have indicated, most of our successful experiences have been accompanied by the stress response. Voila! We have classically conditioned our stress response to success. To the extent that we want success, we trigger our stress response. If our stress response is so valuable and so important to achieving success, why would we want to constrain it?

Well, this is our unconscious position and source of struggle. We are in this incredible catch-22 where, at the same time, stress helps us achieve success and also moves us closer to burnout. Figure 2, on page 54, presents, in graphic form, the relationship between amount of stress or arousal and our level of performance, showing the drop-off with too much stress or nervous system activation. You will also note the second curve labeled "B." As we develop our resilience, we become more resistant to the harmful effects of stress. In fact, there are two ways that increased resilience makes a difference in your life. I refer to both as your "resilience advantage." You will note, as resilience increases, higher levels of stress actually produce higher levels of performance and a wider window of peak performance. In addition, when you are more resilient, you can tolerate higher levels of stress before it harms either your performance or your health.

Problems occur when we lose sight of our optimal level of stress. And most of us never learned how to determine or achieve this optimal level. While stress is good, too much stress is definitely bad. Again, studies have found that beyond a moderate level, stress begins to impair performance. It makes us less capable of thinking creatively and solving problems, and we become distracted. Our thinking becomes stereo-typed, making it difficult to explore new directions.

The most important takeaway from this discussion is not that you should restrict your stress. Instead, I am suggesting that you be more aware of your stress and thus more selective in your choices of when to turn on the stress response. The two operational words here are "selec-tive" and "choices." Selective: you want to be more discriminating as to the situations that activate your stress response and the frequency of that activation. Choice: through following The Path, one goal will be to make your activation of the stress response more within your control rather than a habit that gets triggered indiscriminately.

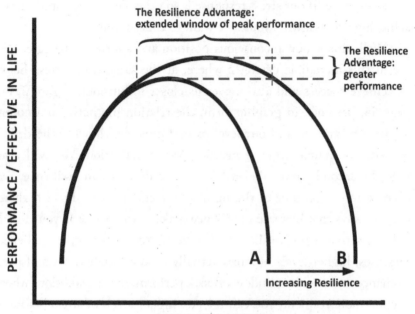

THE RESILIENCE RESPONSE

FIGURE 2 | The relationship between level of arousal and performance and effectiveness in life. The two curves show how increased resilience helps sustain and even improve performance at higher levels of stress and arousal, delaying performance impairment at high levels of stress. I refer to this as the "resilience advantage."

This notion of how we automatically trigger our stress response and the degree to which that is outside of our control, where we are its victims, will be more fully explored in the next chapter. One final word on whether stress is good or bad. Recent research is indicating that one's attitude toward stress can be a factor. People who believe stress is good appear to be less impacted by the stress. Go to The Path and complete steps ten through twelve now.

STEP 10 *There are two aspects to stress that need to be recognized: quality and quantity.*

Quality: Positive stresses, referred to previously as eustress, in general are less harmful to your body than stresses associated with fear, worry, or concern that you may not have the necessary resources to meet demand. For example, time pressures and frustrations fall into this category. There is one other factor that determines the impact of stress. The more you embrace the challenges and stresses of life, the less they will affect you. The more you resist or shrink away from life's challenges, the greater their impact. What is the quality of your stresses?

Quantity: No matter how successful you are, too much stress can become a problem. Is this currently true for you?

Identifying your "good" stresses and your "bad" stresses. Good stress is when you are setting healthy limits and is the result of positive and productive experiences.

Bad stresses are when you are feeling overwhelmed, when the stress continues long after the event and starts long before. Also, when the burden feels as though it's more than you can handle.

STEP 11 *Recognizing how you like stress*

Can you think of ways that you encourage your stress response? For example, if you procrastinate or wait until the last minute to do a task, you are making it more stressful. You might even think you do a better job when you do this. But I've analyzed this impression that many people hold and have determined that it's just an illusion.

STEP 12 *What are your conditioned stress associations?*

If there are people, situations, or places that have caused you distress in the past, a conditioning process may cause them to automatically trigger a stress or danger response, just like Pavlov's bell.

Do you have learned associations that increase your stress? Are there places, situations, or people who—because of your history— create negative expectations and thereby automatically trigger your concern, tension, and stress?

IT'S ALL IN THE EYES OF THE BEHOLDER

Anything that creates a sense of danger or even uncertainty will trigger your stress response and the mobilization of your body's resources and defenses. For this reason, your stress response is open to your particular interpretation of what's dangerous. In other words, stress is subjective; that means that what is stressful to you may not be stressful to another person. It is subject to the interpretation of danger by the person experiencing the event. Thus, if you believe you are in danger, even if the threat is not real, you will trigger your stress response.

This means that your stress response is subject to your particular and individual history. If you learned through your childhood environment that the world is unsafe, you carry this belief, perhaps unconsciously, into your adult life. In new situations your first intuition will be of danger. Before you know it, what your brain and body consider danger signals will trigger a stress response and the expectation that something bad will happen. You will thus be triggering your stress response on a frequent basis. One former client, let's call him Bob, grew up with a parent who could be nice one minute and abusive the next. He lived his life on edge, waiting to see the expression on his parent's face. The first moment was always scary.

The basic message that Bob learned in childhood was that the world and people could be dangerous, and that you never know what to expect. Thus he was always on guard, always cautious, and very sensitive to the facial expressions of others. His stress response was easily triggered because, for him, the world was a dangerous place. What's interesting is that more recent events and experiences, although much more positive and benign, did not change his perspective or expectation. This is because our early childhood experiences have the greatest impact on the developing brain. We will delve into this in more detail in the next chapter, when we explore the impact of childhood learning and adaptation along with its neurological imprint—our primitive Gestalts. The basic message is that our wonderful and necessary ability to adapt gets short-circuited during our childhood "survival learning." Do steps thirteen and fourteen now.

STEP 13   *Your expectations*

When you enter an unfamiliar environment, do you tend to be wary, or are you open and excited about possibilities?

Do you look for what might go right—or what might go wrong?

What are your expectations of others? Are you on guard or more focused on the positive?

Would you say you have "catastrophic expectations" about future events?

Do you come from an open heart, or from protecting your heart?

STEP 14   *Patterns you have difficulty getting out of*

Can you identify your thinking or behavior that you know doesn't serve you but you haven't been able to change?

THE THREE LEVELS OF THE BRAIN AND THE CONSEQUENCES OF TOO MUCH STRESS

Let's take a look at another consequence of the effect of stress. When there is danger, or when you think there is danger, your instinct is to protect yourself or run from the danger. This instinct for self-preservation activates the deepest centers of your brain—the most primitive centers of the midbrain. We have these survival centers in common with reptiles. As we move up the phylogenetic scale (that's a fancy way of saying as we move from the most primitive organisms to the most evolved, meaning us humans), we go through all the intermediate levels. Through the evolutionary process, newer brain areas and brain function overlay the more primitive ones. We have the second level of the brain in common with mammals. This brings in the limbic centers of the brain, which have to do with emotions, behaviors, motivation, and long-term memory. Laid on top of this are the most recent centers, the cortex and the frontal cortex. These are the most complex brain centers and have to do with reasoning and other more advanced cognitive functions.

But when we think there is danger, the lower, more primitive survival centers take over. It's time for fight or flight, not for debating nuances or detail. It's not the time for considering what's beautiful, what's artful. And there certainly isn't time, as far as our survival brain is concerned, for considering a lot of options. What do you think this means? Yes, of course: it means that we don't think too well. We fall into more stereotypical behaviors.

For this reason, when we are engaged in continual fight-or-flight behavior, we are not as good at problem-solving or being creative. We are not as good at being flexible or adaptive and identifying the various options of a situation. In other words, we leap before we look. You may notice this behavior—if not in yourself, certainly in people who surround you: the person who comes to conclusions too quickly, the person who responds in similar ways to very different situations.

YOUR TYPICAL DAY

Are you like many of the people in my workshops? When you awaken in the morning, first you become aware of your anxieties, your worries, or at least, all those things you think about almost automatically that may be of concern. Today's world is an obstacle course of stresses and fears that challenge our ability to cope. This results in an epidemic of chronic illnesses, trauma, and burnout. Success is difficult enough, but achieving success while staying healthy and maintaining a balanced life is difficult but achievable—on The Path. Go to step fifteen now.

STEP 15 *Your typical day*

Think about your typical day. In my workshops, I ask participants to imagine sitting and watching a movie of their day, played before them. Notice how much of the day you spend under pressure. This can be time pressure, decision pressure, or personal interaction discomfort.

It can be financial pressure, and it can be concern over personal health. Many of the people I work with notice that they are jumping from one stressful situation to another in the course of the day. They also discover that they rarely give themselves time to unwind or relax. It is hard for them to take a five-minute break.

This is not a test; it's a first step in an awareness process that will ultimately help you to function more optimally.

As with other steps on The Path, take a neutral stance in this process. You may also have some compassion for yourself if you recognize how much you are pushed around by events.

You are now at the end of chapter three's segment of The Path. Take a moment to appreciate yourself for the effort you are making to become more resilient by recognizing the signposts you have reached.

SIGNPOST

- You have shown gratitude for the fact that your basic survival needs are met.
- You have identified your background stresses.
- You have observed and commented on your stress response.
- You made an assessment of your adaptation energy and reviewed your symptom list.
- You began identifying your stress triggers.
- You have looked at your relationship to stress, including your danger expectations.
- You reviewed your typical day to further notice your stress.

CHAPTER 4

RESISTANCE TO OVERCOMING OLD PATTERNS

Unlocking Your Ability to Adapt

WAKE UP!

If you are going to get onto The Path and stay on The Path, you have to recognize the invisible obstacles that keep getting in your way. To be on The Path, you must learn to have your eyes wide open—to be awake. When you are asleep, metaphorically, you don't know you are asleep. That's the reason you keep making the same mistakes in your life or forgetting to do the very things you know will help you. "What's going on?" you say, as you keep doing the old behavior.

It may be difficult for you to acknowledge that you are asleep with your eyes wide open or living in a partial trance. It may be easier if I refer to this as acting from a habit pattern or automatic behavior that keeps you from being awake or aware. But however I refer to it, the results are the same: You don't have control over your life, and you have difficulty overcoming old patterns that don't serve you. So, the first step in looking at your resistance is to recognize that much of the time you are not awake. If the goal of being on The Path is taking control and responsibility for your life, then you must be "response–able"—and for this, you must wake up!

NEURO-PROCEDURAL PATTERNS INTERFERING WITH AWARENESS

How is it that our brains are capable of doing so many different things at the same time? How are we humans able to engage in more and more complex behavior and thinking? How is it that we can even get out of bed in the morning without having to direct each muscle in our body to do what it needs to lift, stand, and move?

These are examples of the brilliance of the developmental process and the way our brains are organized. It is a process in which our brain clumps learning into procedural memories—functional and interrelated groupings of learned behaviors. With increased experience and connection of a series of behaviors or thoughts, they become linked together in the brain and thus are automatically triggered together when needed. As has been noted by Donald Hebb, a pioneer of brain science, "Neurons that fire together wire together."

It is this organizing principle that allows you to read this page, and these words, without having to read letter by letter. You are able to grasp the meaning of each word and even groupings of words immediately. When you stand up and walk across the room, you do not have to think of each individual muscle activity. In fact, you don't even have to think about the process of walking because it has become automatic and part of procedural memories established long ago in your childhood.

Our brains are designed to respond to novelty, those things that are out of the ordinary, while typically ignoring the more common experiences. The other day I visited a friend who lives near an airport. Shortly after arriving, I was startled by the sound of a jet roaring nearby. *Wow,*

I thought, *that was loud*. After the third or fourth jet interrupted my thoughts, I looked over at my host. I was surprised to note that she was going about her business as usual. I could not detect any awareness of the sounds that were so distracting to me.

What was new and novel to me had become routine and even background sound for her. Her brain had adapted and adjusted, and it allowed her to go about a more or less normal life. This example highlights how we orient and react to new stimuli; once we adjust to these stimuli and determine that there is nothing of importance, our brain pays them no notice.

Similarly, when we first learn new behaviors, we must focus and attend to this new process. But once we've learned the new behaviors, for the most part, we no longer pay attention to them.

This attribute of our brain allows for increased levels of complexity. On an ongoing basis it takes new, learned information and turns it into habits and automatic patterns that free up our awareness or consciousness to focus on new material. A common example of this tendency occurs when we travel a familiar route. Often we arrive at our destination and don't remember any of the details of the trip. We might even comment that our car knows the route and got us to our destination.

While this is a great ability of our brains, it does have its downside. The tendency to look for and even crave the novel can leave us bored with the common. The tendency to take frequently experienced stimuli and place them into procedural memories can result in our reduced ability to focus, to notice and pay attention when we are not jolted by newness and novelty.

This reliance on automatic patterns makes it more difficult to notice habits that need to be changed or adjusted. Our growing tendency to move through our day just as we did yesterday and the day before makes it that much more difficult to do things in a new and better way. This is what I refer to as being "unconscious." Most important, it leaves you less capable of noticing behaviors that are harmful or self-destructive. Take the first two steps on The Path now.

STEP 1 *Identifying a habit*

To be on The Path you need to face your obstacles, be aware, and not hide them from yourself.

Begin to think of and identify habits of yours that you don't like or have tried to change. Habits can be behaviors that don't serve you, such as putting something off for later and then forgetting to do it. They can be habitual ways you talk to yourself and undermine your self-confidence, such as saying, "Boy, am I stupid" when you make a mistake. Or any time you say, "I can't."

When you become aware of a pattern you typically engage in that holds you back, simply notice it without putting yourself down. Being a "witness" is an important step in moving forward on The Path.

STEP 2 *Remembering yourself*

As mentioned in chapter two, Gurdjieff referred to "remembering yourself" as being present to the moment, witnessing yourself. One of the key ingredients to being on The Path is the ability to be present and awake in the moment. But how do we remember to remember?

One way is through the use of cues. We are going to use a common fixture of your environment—the doorway—as your cue to wake up and remember.

Every time you walk through a portal, an entryway, I'd like you to use this cue to "wake up." Simply be a witness to yourself in the moment. In this manner, you will begin your training of being more present and thus "response-able" in life.

GOING AGAINST THE LAWS OF CONDITIONING

When you start out training to become a psychologist, you take many courses focused on theories about behavior. One of the first lessons is that behavior that is reinforced will be strengthened and continued, while behavior that isn't reinforced or that is negatively reinforced will be extinguished. In other words, it will be less and less likely to occur. What this means is that we repeat behaviors that yield the goodies. And we stop engaging in behaviors that either don't give us rewards or that give us pain.

This simple yet elegant concept is what's behind the process of adaptation, making the necessary adjustments in life based on our interaction with our environment. This ability to learn from life's lessons, to continually learn and improve based on experience, can be referred to as adaptability. And we can say that the better we are at this process, the more resilient we are. Adaptation is the hallmark of resilience and optimal performance.

When you recognize the consequences of your behavior, and those consequences are negative, you no longer expect to exhibit that behavior. But noooo. Despite our good intentions and the continual opportunities to learn from our mistakes and life lessons, we find ourselves making the same mistakes over and over again. This, in fact, might be one of the most frustrating experiences in your life.

Whether it's the obvious issues of not getting enough sleep, exercise, and other self-care behavior, or it's keeping your guard up and staying tense when it's safe to let go, you engage in all sorts of behaviors that do not serve your best interests and, in fact, cause harm. In my work with thousands of clients and workshop participants, I consistently encounter people who, despite experiencing the negative consequences of excessive stress, continue to engage in behaviors that trigger the stress response. It is almost as if we "crave" stress even when it's destroying us, as if it were a drug.

And in fact, it does trigger a drug—a natural drug response: adrenaline, to be exact. As strange as it may seem, we can actually become addicted to the release of our own naturally produced chemical. If, for example, you are a person who tends to push down your feelings, you will notice feeling somewhat depressed. I believe that much of depression is simply this pushing down of feelings. Similarly, we might get into a pattern of shallow breathing (reducing oxygen intake and thus becoming less awake) as another way of not noticing feelings. The consequence of these behaviors, the feeling of depression, is sometimes countered by the need for an adrenaline rush. The release of adrenaline, giving us a sense of waking up, simply feels good.

This is only the beginning of a long list of reasons we crave stress and thus have an automatic reluctance to manage it in any way. In addition to being dangerous, it also interferes with the process of adaptation and healthy learning.

WE DON'T TAKE CHANCES WITH OUR SURVIVAL RESPONSE

As we add to the reasons that you resist appropriately managing your stress response and maintaining the condition of optimal balance in your life and body, close to the top of this list is the stress response's position as a survival mechanism. Obviously, nothing else is important if you don't survive. So from the perspective of the hierarchy of what your brain and body focus on, surviving is at the top.

This means that you will not take chances with what you learned, what was "conditioned" during your first years of life—when you were figuring out how the world worked and what was successful in helping you survive. As I've mentioned previously, your world, and your training ground, was your childhood environment.

So your life lessons got locked in as survival responses under those conditions. And now there is a part of you that doesn't want to let go, because it believes your survival, and possibly your success, is dependent on those obsolete lessons. Make sure you go to The Path for steps three, four, and five.

STEP 3   *In the moment*

Some of you will sit down and eat a meal, perhaps one that is delicious, and not pay attention to the taste of the food, finishing the meal before you know it. Here is one common activity we all engage in: we usually eat three times each day.

Over the next few days, pay more attention to the taste of your food. See if you can enjoy the process of eating and being present.

STEP 4 *What are some of the lessons of life you are ignoring?*

These lessons may be in your relationships or in your professional life.

For example, you may have a friend or partner who demonstrates trustworthiness, but instead of letting down your guard with this person, you act as if he or she might hurt you or be critical of you. This is a lesson learned from your childhood.

In general, you might be safer than you are willing to acknowledge.

Or you might be exhibiting low self-confidence, another lesson from childhood, while ignoring and not adjusting your self-image to the successes of more recent years.

STEP 5 *What are the lessons of YOUR childhood?*

What are the messages that have gotten imprinted in you—deeply in you—that perhaps guide you in the wrong direction? Examples of this might be: "I can't rely on anyone," "Don't let down my guard; it's dangerous," "There is something wrong with me; I'm not OK," "I'm not lovable."

IF OUR STRESS RESPONSE IS GOOD, THEN MORE IS BETTER

I have already listed the many ways that your stress response serves you, mobilizes you to take action, helps you focus and be more motivated. It enhances performance. There is great reluctance, therefore, to set any limit on something you feel is helpful or needed. Thus, the word "management" itself tends to turn you off. Frequently, I hear someone I'm working with voice the fear that if they try to relax, they might become lazy or unproductive. Many people believe there is a slippery slope: start relaxing a little, and pretty soon you will find it difficult to do any work. For others, part of their stress is the fear of their life falling apart.

Under these circumstances, they can only think of hanging on, even if it means maintaining high stress and tension levels. For these people, there's great discomfort with letting go and being vulnerable.

I have also explained how it is a survival mechanism. It's a protective response, like circling the wagons and putting up the wall. But this isn't a case where if something is good, then more is better. You can have too much of a good thing. And when there is too much, it's no longer good. Notice your frustration when more exertion is not getting you closer to your goal.

This is most evident in my work with elite athletes. When the stress response, or the activation of the body, goes too far, the results are immediate and obvious. You notice it in the final minutes of an important basketball game, when a free throw clanks against the front rim of the basket. This is a clear indication that the tension in the ballplayer's arm muscles was too tight, restricting the appropriate flexion and extension of the arm. It was also true for a tennis player I worked with who, in big matches, would cramp partway through the game.

Once you have reached an optimal level of arousal, you can perform at your best. You don't require additional energy or tension to perform any better. In fact, any additional activation will only interfere with your best performance and fatigue you faster—prematurely draining the resources of your body. When this process continues over a period of time, you begin to experience a breakdown, with symptoms that may include headaches, stomachaches, insomnia, high blood pressure, and, ultimately, burnout. Check out step six on The Path now.

STEP 6 *Identifying ways in your life that you keep the stress response going beyond its usefulness*

You may worry about an event that will take place a day in the future, triggering the stress response for a full twenty-four hours instead of just the hour of the event.

Or, after you complete a performance or a difficult interaction with another person, you worry about how you did and what will happen, thus keeping your stress response activated long after its usefulness. What ways can you identify that amplify your stress response?

MEETING EMOTIONAL NEEDS

It is instructive to observe the person who has plenty of money and all he or she could want yet who places himself or herself under continual stress. By examining an extreme example, we may shed light on our own behavior. Take the executive who couldn't just sit and read on his day off. Whenever he did that, he felt uncomfortable, as though he were doing something wrong. Another executive, referred after a quadruple bypass heart surgery, was back at his fourteen-hour day as a producer six months later. As we examined this behavior, he realized that the only way he could allow himself to stop working was if he were in a hospital bed.

For most of you this would appear extreme; yet on closer examination, you might also find it difficult to slow down or take time to simply relax during your day. These are different forms of "I must be productive to feel good about myself." Most of my clients find it difficult to take ten to fifteen minutes out of their day to practice a relaxation exercise—something you will be asked to do as part of being on The Path.

Many of our emotional needs and our self-worth are tied to our performance and our accomplishments. We are more concerned about what others think and feel than about our own sense of self. Thus we are driven by the need for the approval or acceptance of others. You will be addressing this issue in much greater depth in the sixth pillar of resilience. For the moment, it's sufficient to begin identifying examples of this in your life. Go to step seven on The Path now.

STEP 7   *Noticing how your emotional needs impact your behavior*

We are on the part of The Path focused on self-observation and awareness and, as noted previously, being witness to your own patterns.

Think about how your emotional needs determine your behavior.

For example, do you have difficulty saying no to people's requests for fear of being rejected, incurring anger, or upsetting someone else? Or, to keep proving your worth, do you push yourself a bit further than you feel comfortable or know is good for you? What's true for you?

EMOTIONS CAN BE UNCOMFORTABLE AND, WELL, MESSY

There is a simple device called a galvanic skin response meter. It measures the moisture on the surface of your skin. You may notice at times that when you are anxious, your hands become moist or clammy. It may occur before a test or before a performance. Conversely, when you relax, your hands become drier.

This phenomenon demonstrates the extraordinary mechanisms that keep the body in balance. This is how it works: When there is danger, a challenge, or simply uncertainty, your body mobilizes by triggering the stress response, as noted in a previous chapter. When the body mobilizes for fight or flight, when your heart speeds up and muscles brace for action, your body is actually working like a factory to produce more energy. Every cell in your body, in fact, is like a tiny factory working to produce energy. It metabolizes sugars for this purpose.

Like any factory, one of the byproducts of the production of energy is heat. Homeostasis is the process whereby your body is always monitoring levels: levels of blood pressure, levels of heart rate, levels of blood sugar, and levels of body temperature. Its mission is to keep all these levels . . . well . . . level within a very narrow "safe" range. When any system starts to move out of this range, the body tries to restore the optimal level. Among those things, the body has to maintain a safe level of internal temperature, the body's core temperature.

When fight or flight activates the body and burns fuel for this activation, the skin turns into a giant radiator. The pores of the skin open and release moisture. When the moisture hits the air and evaporates, it cools the body back into its optimal range.

With a galvanic skin response meter, you can measure the level of moisture—actually, you send a very tiny current from one finger to the next. The more moisture (in other words, the greater the stress response), the lower the resistance in the electrical circuit and the higher the pitch of the tone that the device creates. With relaxation and a reduction in moisture, there is a higher resistance in the circuit, and the tone goes down—it decreases pitch. This is the basis of biofeedback. This device lets you know immediately when you do something that helps you relax, as you will hear the tone go down. Conversely, it will let you know whenever you become tense, as the sound will go up. This feedback process speeds up the learning of self-regulation.

One of the strange things that happens when someone is using this device as a biofeedback tool to relax is that the sound will be going down as the person is going deeper into relaxation, and suddenly, there will be a slight jolt and the sound will bounce back up. This occurs because subjects get to a point in the relaxation process where they suddenly feel something that makes them uncomfortable, such that they become a bit activated, sending the biofeedback sound back up.

If we continue with the relaxation process, the sound will reverse and come down again. But here is the interesting thing: as they get to the same point in the relaxation process, the same jolt will occur, sending activation and sound back up.

What is going on here? Why, as they are in the midst of relaxing, would this occur? The answer is that as they relax, they get to a point of calm where ignored or pushed-down emotions begin coming to the surface, making them uncomfortable and triggering this activation. Most of the time, they, and many of you, are so engaged in the outside world,

the world of stress, that these feelings—unfinished business from yesterday, last month, or years ago—are kept at bay. They are camouflaged
by busyness—until you try to relax! In other words, your discomfort
with emotions can help to maintain stress as a distraction from these
feelings and make it difficult to relax and be calm. Go to step eight on
The Path now.

STEP 8   *This can be a sensitive topic—the avoidance and accumulation
of unfinished emotional business.*

If you have developed really good means of disregarding and not being
aware of this area of your life, like being asleep, how can you even
recognize it? We will delve more deeply into this issue when we work
on resilience component number six: emotional balance and mastery.
For right now, let's pick the low-hanging fruit and identify what you do
notice about your unfinished business.

What feelings and emotions might you be ignoring by staying activated, stressed, or simply busy all of the time? What unfinished business do you have, and with which people, that it might be easier not to
notice? Husband, wife, or partner? Parents? Children? Colleague, boss,
or supervisor? Even if you believe it's more trouble trying to resolve
these feelings, not achieving resolution causes these emotions to go
underground and affect you unconsciously.

I'm not implying that these issues are going totally unrecognized,
but that by keeping activated, you are not constantly faced with feelings
you have not found a way of resolving.

THE STRESS RESPONSE HELPS YOU FEEL ALIVE

If you have found ways of ignoring your feelings—and we all do this—
then a likely consequence is that, to some extent, you have numbed yourself. You see, you are not able to selectively make yourself unaware of
only negative feelings! When you depress or push down your anger, or

unconsciously engage in shallow breathing to numb yourself not to notice sadness, you are numbing yourself to all feelings, even the good ones.

If you try to not notice through dissociation—the process of distracting yourself from the moment—or by any other means, this does not just take place in your head. Your entire body needs to collude in this masquerade. And what your body typically does is clamp down, tighten, or otherwise constrict in order to hold in the feeling. This process was referred to as "armoring" by Wilhelm Reich, a brilliant psychiatrist writing in the middle of the twentieth century. He, Alexander Lowen, and other "body psychologists" referred to what happens physically when you ignore your feelings. The result is that your body loses some of its vitality and ability to fully function, to flow, to fully feel, including the ability to fully feel joy.

How do you cope with this loss of aliveness? Or, perhaps it's better said like this: How do you compensate for this loss of awareness and loss of feeling? A convenient way is to trigger the stress response and send adrenaline coursing through the body to wake up and feel alive. Go to step nine on The Path now.

STEP 9 *How have you noticed your reduced capacity to fully feel joy?*

It might be the occasional—or not so occasional—sense of depression. It might be some disappointment in not feeling how you would expect to feel after something positive occurs. It might be a loss of interest in activities that used to give you pleasure. How do you notice decreased joy in your life?

LOYALTY TO PARENTS WHO DIDN'T HAVE A HANDLE ON STRESS OR THEIR EMOTIONS

Nobel laureate Konrad Lorenz conducted a very famous series of experiments in the middle of the twentieth century. He found that if he hung out with eggs of goslings and ducks and then was the first object that these ducklings and goslings observed when they hatched, they would bond to him as the first moving object they encountered. This bonding seemed to form immediately and appeared to be irreversible.

The process of learning is supposed to be either forgettable or modifiable, depending on new information and experience. But this bonding, or "imprinting," as it was called, was so permanent that even at maturity, these animals tried to court and attempted to mate with humans if they were imprinted to them. Robert Firestone refers to this in his appropriately named book, *The Fantasy Bond*, in which we hold on to a fantasy about our first relationships in order to maintain a sense of connection.

In your own developmental process, you not only become imprinted with your primary caregivers but with their approach to life, including how they handle problems and stress. A strange sense of loyalty might occur, in which you feel compelled, without even knowing it, to follow some of the inappropriate patterns of your mother and/or father. You then feel like you are betraying them if you try to do it differently or better. Go to step ten on The Path now.

STEP 10　*Recognizing lessons of childhood*

See if you can identify some of the ways that you are stuck in patterns of your parents. It might be a sense of disorganization or it might be the way you deal with frustration or anger. For example, you might feel it's not OK to express anger or to cry.

It may be how you associate with the wrong types of people—people who are critical or who otherwise don't serve your best interests.

How are you following in their footsteps?

CONDITIONED ASSOCIATIONS TO SUCCESS AND RELIEF

I had a client, and she is not unique, who would always worry when taking an exam. She would worry before the exam, when taking the exam, and then afterward she would worry that she did poorly. I asked her, "How poorly did you do in all your tests?" "I always got "As," she responded to me. *Hmm,* I thought, *always worried and always got As.*

There were actually two very interesting facts about this: First was that despite all of her successes and their consistency, she never learned to expect success. In other words, her old beliefs withstood years of contrary experience and positive reinforcement. Her success certainly didn't "go to her head."

And secondly, and this is what's relevant here, I realized that a strange pairing took place. Remember the comments of Dr. Hebb, "Neurons that fire together wire together"? Here we can see that the neurons firing along with worry and tension, as the client prepared for an exam, were constantly and consistently paired with the wiring associated with a successful result, getting an A. In other words, this client, and many others, learned, without being aware, that whenever she was worried, anxious, or stressed, she was successful!

It's interesting to think that this same concept can be applied to procrastination, such as the person who says, "I do best when I wait until the last minute." I would suggest that what is happening here is a similar pairing of procrastination with relief at completing a task.

The bottom line is that some of our most ineffective behaviors get inadvertently associated with success and thus get wired with the success. We then tend to keep repeating this behavior, even though it is not responsible for our success, but in fact, our success may be accomplished in spite of this behavior. In psychology this is referred to as "superstitious behavior." Go to step eleven on The Path now.

STEP 11 *Identifying some of your own superstitious behaviors*

Can you think of how some of your worry or anxiety has become associated with success? And what about procrastination? Does it really serve you?

CONCLUSIONS

When you started this chapter, I'm sure you did not realize all the hidden obstacles to becoming resilient. But this was not meant to discourage you or overwhelm you. Instead it was to help you in the process of becoming more aware, which in fact places you on The Path. So even though I am identifying, and you are learning about, many obstacles, this process is putting you squarely in the middle of The Path. Good luck as you continue to follow it.

SIGNPOST

- You have become more aware of habits that don't serve you.
- You have taken time to "remember yourself" by using doorways, or portals, as cues.
- You have noticed your overuse of the stress response when it doesn't serve you.
- You have become aware of your difficulty taking time to fully relax.
- You have noticed your avoidance of feelings and your unfinished emotional business.
- You have noticed your patterns that were learned from your parents.

CHAPTER 5

TAPPING IN TO NEUROPLASTICITY
New Brain Growth, New Possibilities,
Creativity, and New Models of Change

What I love about science is that you never know what you're going to find around the next bend. You never know what new discovery can potentially turn the world upside down by showing a new and totally unexpected perspective. This has certainly been the case in our understanding of the brain. When I first began my training as a psychologist, the common belief in neuroscience was that we are born with a full complement of brain cells. As we grow up and age, these brain cells slowly die off and are not replaced. In other words, at birth we had more brain cells than we would ever have again; thus, in a sense, it was downhill from there.

Early in my career, I had the privilege of studying as a postdoctoral fellow in the laboratory of James McGaugh. He was studying the neuroscience of learning and memory at the University of California, Irvine, in 1971. At the time, the Department of Psychobiology was a hotbed of exciting new research. I was able to walk down the hallways and open doors that let me into new areas of brain research. One of these doors opened into the laboratory of Gary Lynch. I remember Gary—a wiry-haired mad scientist—being very excited about his new findings.

His research, along with that of his colleague, Carl Cotman, was challenging this notion that throughout our life span, even during childhood, we continually lost but never gained new nerve cells. My own research was centered on a small area of the brain called the hip-pocampus. This area of the brain was believed to be involved in memory. By placing very tiny electrodes into the hippocampus (in rats), I was learning about how that area of the brain functions and, more specifically, how it was involved in the process of learning and memory.

Gary was doing studies in which he lesioned small areas of the brain and then observed what happened. What he discovered was that nerve cells in areas adjacent to the lesioned area began developing new dendrites, or nerve cell extensions, that grew into the areas of lesion. Later research confirmed that these new dendrites were functional.

Subsequent research in this as well as from other laboratories around the world—and with the advent of brain imaging—have found more and more evidence of new nerve growth. We now know that musicians, for example, show specific growth associated with many hours of practicing and using their hands. For example, the area of the brain associated with motor control of the left fingers is much larger in a violinist than in the average person. Blind individuals who have been using the technique of Braille, in which their fingers move across a page with raised letters to actually "read" with their fingers, will have expanded the areas of the brain devoted to sensing with these fingers. These were early signs of the brain's neuroplasticity.

In the past twenty years, research in this field has exploded. A great deal of new information has been discovered about how the brain works. We now know, contrary to the beliefs held for hundreds of years, that we are not born with a full complement of nerve cells that we lose over time. Instead, the brain is capable of birthing new nerve cells throughout our lives. This process, called "neurogenesis," can be triggered in as brief as a thirty-minute experience. With appropriate intentions, goals, and a specific plan of action, such as The Path, it is possible to enhance this process of neurodevelopment and make significant positive changes in your brain—and thus in your behavior and your life.

NEUROGENESIS AND RESILIENCE

I have defined resilience from many different perspectives thus far: It's the ability to bounce back, or as I prefer to say, bounce forward; it's optimal self-regulation and adaptability; it's being aware or awake for as many moments in your life as possible. Here is another aspect of resilience: It's the optimal birthing of new nerve cells—or brain cells. Using words such as "birth" and "new" even sounds resilient. They signify something growing, emerging, regenerating, becoming, trans-forming. They indicate that depletion and damage can be overcome by new growth. The good news is that you, too, can get in on this action!

Your brain's capability for neurogenesis is an important aspect of being resilient. How you address this aspect of yourself will help deter-mine your resilience. And here again I come back to this little area of the brain, the hippocampus, that I became so intimate with during my early research.

HIPPOCAMPUS, STRESS, AND RESILIENCE

You now are becoming an expert on the stress response. Yes, you need it, you want it, and you are beginning to realize that you also need to exert some mastery over it. Here is another piece of the puzzle: The hippocampus, that beautiful little brain nucleus I studied years ago, plays an intimate role in resilience. When you activate your body, and your nervous system goes into action, and when your cardiovascular system revs up, speeding up your heart and your blood pressure, it's the hippocampus that sends a message to turn down this autonomic nervous system activation. Yes, the hippocampus modulates heart rate and autonomic function by applying the brake to the stress response. It helps us "chill out." Chronic stress causes atrophy and dysfunction of the hippocampus. When this occurs, it reduces your capacity to dampen the stress response and your ability to relax.

If this weren't enough reason to appreciate and be concerned about this little corner of the brain, here in this tiny nucleus is where much of neurogenesis takes place. The hippocampus is a hotbed—or rather, a nursery—for new nerve cell birthing and growth. We want it to function well. It turns out that chronic stress has another significant negative impact. It reduces and can completely eliminate neurogenesis in the hippocampus.

Other ways that impairment of the hippocampus affects us is its reduced ability to release the neurotransmitter dopamine and modulate pain. Neurotransmitters are magical neurochemicals, meaning that they are chemicals we find in the brain and nervous system. Dopamine is of primary importance among these very important elements. It drives our behavior and our motivations. It modulates endogenous opiate (opiate-like substances created in the brain) action to help reduce your experience of pain. We know, for example, that people diagnosed with fibromyalgia—a chronic pain condition that reduces resilience—have a damaged hippocampus. These patients' experience of pain, fatigue, and stiffness are directly related to reduced integrity of the hippocampus.

FOUR TYPES OF NEUROGENESIS

I suggest that there are four levels or types of neurogenesis. At the first level, the birthing of new brain cells occurs even when you are engaged in habitual behaviors. Even when there is nothing new in your life and new learning isn't occurring, your brain is still birthing new nerve cells. But these new nerve cells will only strengthen existing habit patterns. The new brain cells will fall into place with existing cell assemblies or brain circuits. Thus, the more you engage in old habits, the more you reinforce these patterns.

FOLLOWING YOUR CHILDHOOD BLUEPRINT

At the second level, when you are engaged in learning something new, this new learning will be accompanied by what neuroscientists refer to as "long-term potentiation." This is a fancy term that means structural change is taking place in the brain cells and circuits that are involved with successful behavior change so that it's easier for future signals to pass through this circuit. A building process is taking place; nerve cells are growing new dendritic spines that create more connections with adjacent nerve cells. This is the brain changing to accommodate new learning.

In this case, when neurogenesis takes place and new nerve cells are born, they will carry this new information. In other words, the neurogenesis process captures these changes. In addition, these new nerve cells will also incorporate the new cell assemblies—those new brain circuits that have resulted from the new learned associations.

But even in this example of new learning, the new nerve growth still follows the existing blueprint of your brain. This blueprint is laid down as the foundation of your primitive Gestalt.

This is why your early childhood development and learning have a lifelong impact on your behavior, on your psychology, and on your potential for growth. Childhood lessons such as "I'm not OK," "The world is dangerous," and "You can't trust anybody" establish "growth lines" for new learning and the process of neurogenesis. For example, let's take the childhood lesson of "not being smart enough." This may have been created as a result of poor attention, it may have occurred because your development was slow and you were just a little bit behind other children, it may have happened because your environment was so difficult or scary that you closed down, or it may have developed as a result of the critical messages—or lack of messages—you got from parents or teachers.

Your mother or father may have thought that anything other than an A was bad, giving you the inaccurate message of not being smart if you got a B+ (as was the case with a number of people I've worked with). Or perhaps your parents were too distracted and stressed themselves even to comment on your schoolwork, leaving you to assume their lack of reaction was because you didn't do well enough. Neglect or excessive criticism may have left you with inaccurate messages.

As you grew up and experienced success, instead of taking in this new information and adjusting your self-evaluation, you dismissed the new information as not counting or as not being accurate because it did not match the belief already lodged in your brain and body. It didn't fit with your existing primitive Gestalt brain cell assembly. This is why we frequently hear comments such as "It was luck," "It was coincidence," or "Anybody could've done it" to explain away a good performance or a success. On the other hand, a mistake or poor performance becomes more validation of the old messages and reinforces the primitive Gestalt brain circuits. Thus, our new growth and learning take a predictable path along the lines set out in our childhood. Go to The Path and complete steps one through five.

STEP 1 *Identifying a childhood pattern*

Take a few moments to identify a childhood lesson or pattern that has been difficult for you to get beyond.

Think about it in as much detail as possible. To help you with this, imagine the spokesperson of your primitive Gestalt—your internal voice or internal parent—and imagine this part of yourself reminding you about this lesson. For example, "Remember, don't get too relaxed," "You may not be able to do it," "Don't trust or expect too much," or "It won't last."

STEP 2 *What is the impact?*

How has this pattern held you back? How has it created unnecessary guarding, procrastination, worry, or a reluctance to move forward in your life or career for fear of judgment or rejection? Or perhaps it's put more pressure and stress on you, as you continually try to be or do more.

STEP 3 *What are some of your negative messages?*

What are some of the messages that your internal voice—your old internal parent—gives you that are abusive or negative and that you buy into, despite your awareness? Messages such as "You don't deserve" or "You're not good enough."

In what ways do those messages make you feel inadequate? They may include being hard on yourself or not giving yourself enough credit for your successes and hard work. It might be that you are still punishing yourself for a past mistake.

STEP 4 *Identifying behaviors that hold you back*

What relationships and environments do you maintain that may not be the healthiest for you?

STEP 5 *How do they harm you?*

How might unhealthy relationships and environments be hurting you? For example, you might be in a relationship with a friend who is insecure. As a result, that individual might feel threatened by any success on your part. He or she may not be happy or supportive of your positive steps, even if the individual does not acknowledge this.

One of my clients related a story about growing up in New York. One day in winter when he was twelve, he awoke, looked out his window, and saw all white. A blizzard had already dumped eighteen inches of snow on the ground. This was rare, and it was great. He jumped out of bed and ran downstairs, hopeful that there was enough snow to cancel school for the day. And indeed, school was canceled. "Hallelujah," he cried.

My client, Mike, had a plan. He enjoyed building model airplanes and had set his sights on one particular, extravagant B-52 model. This was his chance to make enough money to buy it. He gobbled down his breakfast, got dressed, put on his heaviest coat and galoshes, grabbed his father's snow shovel, and ran outside. After shoveling his own walkway, he began going door to door asking neighbors if they would like their walkway shoveled for only a dollar. This was his big day.

He worked hard all day, continuing even when he wanted to stop. When he finished his day, he pulled out his wad of one-dollar bills and was very excited and proud of himself. He couldn't wait to get home and show his father. He walked in the door, ran up to his father, and pulled out his earnings. "Look, Dad," he said with a big smile on his face. His father looked at him and said the words that became branded in his head for years to come: "Don't get too big for your britches, son." My client walked away, crestfallen and hurt. After that moment, it became difficult for Mike to fully own his achievements, afraid of being "too big for his britches"—but never realizing, until our session, that this was the reason behind his behavior.

Thus, we continually dismiss information that does not match our childhood training, lessons, and the beliefs our childhood set up. This keeps us stuck in our primitive Gestalts. Most of neurogenesis follows this pattern of keeping within the boundaries set by early learning. As a result, most of the time your brilliance simply goes into gilding your cage. And neurogenesis, new nerve cell birth, and dendritic extensions stay within their established boundaries as you remain loyal to childhood lessons. Another way of saying this is that your ability to adapt has been frozen in the lessons of childhood.

It is important to note that I'm not only referring to childhood lessons and thinking patterns. Emotions and feelings are also part of our primitive Gestalts. Many of these feelings were created even before we had words to describe them. This makes them all the more powerful because, unlike our thinking, they are more difficult to address or argue with. Instead, these feelings, which get easily triggered and are real—although based on old experiences—cause us to scan our present environment searching for a cause for the feeling. In this manner we are continually validating old feelings and old messages by making an inappropriate connection or attribution with something in our present life. And new nerve cell development falls into line with these old primitive Gestalt messages. Again, an example of frozen adaptation.

WHEN NEUROGENESIS FACILITATES RESILIENCE AND OPTIMAL ADAPTATION

The third level of neurogenesis takes place when learning is not constrained by old patterns, by an inaccurate perspective of your world or yourself. It occurs when you are able to shift from an inner voice dominated by the beliefs and internalized messages of your childhood to a healthy internal guidance system; when you are able to make the discrimination between a reaction that is relevant to a current situation and a reaction that is embedded in your primitive Gestalt—in other words, when you are reacting to childhood or old messages.

When you are open to new ways of perceiving and experiencing that don't have to fit your old lessons, then you are beginning to break out of boundaries that constrain your development. That's when a new type of neurogenesis, level three, can take place. This is the level associated with resilience and restored healthy adaptation. Here is where you will enter The Path. When you are open to a new belief, to a new way that things might be, you stimulate a new type of growth and development. You also reinvigorate or reboot your own process of optimal adaptation that childhood learning has interfered with. This is when you are able to benefit most from the lessons of life. You become a peak performer on The Path. Go to steps six and seven on The Path now.

STEP 6   *Speaking from your healthy voice*

In chapter two you began identifying the healthy part of you that wants to achieve success, that wants good things for yourself and that—at its foundation—loves, supports, and accepts you. I'm not suggesting that you have fully embraced this part.

It might still be a very tiny seedling poking its first leaves out of the ground. It might have some tough times ahead.

It might be trying to grow between the cracks of a concrete sidewalk! But its voice, however small, is audible. It might be a whisper; but if you try hard, you can hear it.

This whisper, this seedling, is represented in new nerve cells and new cell assemblies in your brain.

Right now, let's grow some new nerve cells and strengthen these new brain patterns. Let's guide your gene expression: Have this healthy voice speak to you now about the old pattern. Allow this voice to respond to the primitive Gestalt spokesperson by suggesting that while you needed this old pattern during your childhood—to help you get by and survive—it no longer serves you.

With each word and sentence you muster to counter the old voice, you are guiding your genetic expression into constructive new brain growth! Have this new, healthy voice speak up and tell you that you are OK. Even if you make mistakes, you are still OK. And it's time to forgive yourself for whatever you are still blaming yourself about from the past. Again, right now, give yourself some positive messages.

STEP 7 *Imagine hearing a supportive voice*

If you are having difficulty, imagine a good friend of yours, or perhaps a relative, who truly loves you and wants good things for you.

Imagine what they would say right now, and allow that voice to amplify your own weak response.

CREATING YOUR NEW REALITY AND A NEW STORY FOR YOURSELF

You go through life making certain changes to your behaviors and thinking. But some patterns are much more difficult to modify. As mentioned earlier, your blueprint for development has been set in place, and new growth occurs along predicted lines. Your primitive Gestalt pattern, wired into your brain and body, resists significant and real change.

As you might suspect, this discussion is leading you toward the good news: These well-entrenched patterns are susceptible to change. Larry Feig, a neuroscientist at Tufts University School of Medicine in Boston, conducted a study using mice genetically engineered to have memory problems. This means that the memory problems of these mice are hardwired into their genes and into their neurons. The researchers took these memory-deficient mice and raised them in an enriched environment, with toys, exercise, and social interaction for two weeks during their adolescence. The animals' memories improved, which shows that enrichment can boost brain function, even when this would seem impossible based on their genetics.

Even more interesting, these researchers also looked at the molecular correlates of memory called long-term potentiation, or LTP, the biological mechanism that strengthens connections between neurons and is believed to be an important process of memory formation. What they discovered was that the environmental enrichment actually fixed faulty LTP in mice with genetic defects. I hope you recognize the significance of this finding: even genetic impairments, let alone learned brain patterns (your primitive Gestalts), can be repaired!

These mice, after the two-week period in the enriched environment, were returned to a normal environment where they grew up and had off-spring. The next generation of mice also had better memories, despite their genetic defect and never being exposed to the enriched environment. When the brains of these offspring were examined, researchers discovered that the fixed LTP was passed on to the next generation of mice. These findings held true even when the pups were raised by memory-deficient mice that had never had the benefit of toys and social interaction.

This research demonstrates the possibilities—no, the realities—of neuroplasticity. It demonstrates the possibilities for healing from painful childhood training and wounding, and it leaves us with a very powerful conclusion. Choosing new thinking patterns, choosing healthier and enriching environments, and nurturing a new perspective and a new belief system (a new story) can fundamentally restructure your brain. It can heal and repair the lessons and damage of your childhood experiences! It will enhance resilience and peak performance.

GENE EXPRESSION

Neurogenesis involves the process of gene expression. Gene expression is the most fundamental level at which the genotype (your genetic materials) is translated into the phenotype (the behaviors and physical characteristics that you recognize as who you are). What this means is that your genetic code, stored in your DNA or genetic material, is "interpreted" through the process of gene expression.

The brain is capable of birthing new nerve cells, and it can happen quite rapidly. In fact, some types of gene expression (triggering of new nerve cell growth) can occur in just minutes.

Think about the learning that a baby or toddler experiences. Everything in his or her world is new and unique. Let's take a specific example: The first time children hold a fork, they will examine every aspect of it, its prongs, its handle. They will try to use it to hit the food, to push the food, to poke the food. They will be engrossed in the experience and what each of their behaviors produces.

Their focus, engrossment, and interest in the outcome make them "learning machines." Right now I'd like to turn you into a "learning machine." Go to steps eight and nine on The Path.

STEP 8   *Supporting self-acceptance*

This step involves creating a similar attitude of engrossment, wonder, and openness. Children don't approach learning with an already determined perspective of what can or cannot be. They are open to learning a new lesson. So, this step asks you to be interested and open to the lesson being taught.

Let's take just one of the messages of your developing healthy internal voice: "Accept where you are." This message of acceptance is a primary and universal message that we all desire and all deserve. When you come from this perspective, it makes learning and growth much more possible.

Remember, it doesn't mean you are perfect, and it doesn't mean you are at the end point of your development or growth. It simply puts you in harmony with reality—acknowledging "what is" in terms of your development and letting it be OK, rather than allowing it to upset you and put yourself down. The child playing with their fork isn't hampered by worrying that they aren't doing it right.

It thus places you at what I would refer to as a baseline, an acceptable starting point—not in some sort of hole you need to dig yourself out of! (That's what happens when you don't accept what is.)

Now—with interest, excitement, and engrossment—take the position of your developing, healthy, internal voice and tell yourself that you are OK, that the place you are at—warts and all—is acceptable and is the only place you can be right now. Imagine being very young, so that you can re-create the sense of newness of the message, as well as connect with the excitement and passion that a child would experience in learning something new—in this case, that you are OK and that it's important to accept the place you are at now.

Come on, play this game with me—it will create the brain conditions for optimally taking in this message. Not only that, but recognize that this new perspective—that you are OK—is a necessity; it's necessary to break free from your early childhood learning. It will help you reboot your ability to learn and adapt.

STEP 9   *Hearing the positive message from your healthy internal parent*
Throughout the day today (find some way to remind yourself to remember), connect with this new, healthy, internal parent or voice; allow

yourself to play the game of newness, just as if you were a child; hear this message, breathe, and take it in: "I am accepting myself the way I am, warts and all." And notice if this lifts your spirits.

It turns out that this process of gene expression is influenced by many factors. In fact, there is a new area of research called "psychosocial genomics." This discipline studies how the subjective experiences of human consciousness and behavior, along with social dynamics, modulate the process of gene expression. In other words, learning, perception, and how we experience the world contribute to how our genetic material gets transformed during gene expression to create our physical characteristics and our behavior, thinking, and emotions. Gene expression is not preordained!

In his book *The Psychobiology of Gene Expression*, Dr. Ernest Rossi says, "The regulation of gene expression by social factors makes all bodily functions, including all functions of the brain, susceptible to social influences." I will add to this: All these functions are also susceptible to your own subjective perspective—your interpretations— and the personal story you tell about yourself. We can translate this into your real-life situation to recognize that how you treat yourself, how you talk to yourself and about yourself, will influence the ongoing expression of your genetic material. This in turn will determine your personal psychology (and even your biology). If you hold on to the story from your childhood, it will continue to maintain gene expression in old patterns. If you open to a new story—well, what do you think could happen?

Your social interactions—whom you choose as friends and associates, and your social environment—will also have a major impact on your gene expression and your psychology. You can see how much is in your hands and in your control right here and right now. Go to steps ten, eleven, and twelve on The Path.

STEP 10 *Creating a new and supportive story*

Your old pattern, your primitive Gestalt, is based on an old story. I'd like to begin creating a new story, one that I suggest is more accurate.

Please take what you can from it, whatever seems to fit. The new story: You did what you had to do growing up in order to survive and to ensure that your needs would be met. In addition, you learned ways to protect yourself emotionally by developing defensive patterns to manage, ignore, and bury painful feelings.

You did a very good job to protect and survive to get to this point in your life. You also made sacrifices, blaming yourself when your mother or father were unresponsive or abusive in order to keep them in good standing. You did this, too, to maintain the hope that, if you got it right, if you figured out their needs and what they wanted, they would give you the love you needed and deserved.

STEP 11 *Dress rehearsal for a better life*

Visualization—which, in this case, is a dress rehearsal for what you want to happen—can be used now to instigate neurogenesis along new lines of development. Take a few breaths and feel yourself relaxing.

Visualize yourself already accepting a new story and new perspective: that you are OK, that you are a special person with your own unique ways of doing things. Remember, we are visualizing, so for some of you to picture this, you might have to really reach inside and be creative. In this visualization, you are deserving of good things happening to you.

You take care of yourself and are always looking for the best way of interacting with the environment to get your needs met and to achieve success. It is important to realize that no matter what your goals are, no matter what you want for yourself, this new story—this visualized reality—is the most effective way to achieve whatever represents your definition of success!

Appreciate your newfound positive perspective

Accept and appreciate: Give yourself a few minutes now to fully take in and accept these images. Allow yourself to appreciate being in this very positive place for the moment.

THE FOURTH LEVEL: DAVID BOHM AND THE IMPLICATE ORDER

In recent years, discoveries in quantum physics have challenged our view of reality. For example, I can't turn on a switch in my office that causes something else to happen far away, such as turning on a light bulb, without a direct connection, such as a signal the switch sends to the bulb. But we now have evidence that what is referred to as "non-locality" or "action at a distance" is possible. An example of this is the finding that when two electrons—the negatively charged particles orbiting the center of an atom—are separated by great distances, they can still communicate: When one changes orientation in a certain way, the other electron makes the same adjustment simultaneously. A connection exists that defies our current rules of reality in the form of basic physical laws.

David Bohm was a pioneer in the interpretation of these new concepts and their implications. In 1952, the year after a series of discussions with Albert Einstein, Bohm published two papers sketching what later came to be called the causal interpretation of quantum theory—which, he said, "opens the door for the creative operation of underlying, and yet subtler, levels of reality."

In his view, subatomic particles such as electrons are not simple, structureless particles, but highly complex, dynamic entities. He rejects the view that their motion is fundamentally uncertain or ambiguous. They follow a precise path—one determined not only by conventional physical forces but also by a more subtle force that Bohm calls the "quantum potential." The quantum potential guides the motion of particles by providing "active information" about the whole environment. Bohm gives the analogy of a ship being guided by radar signals: the radar carries information from all around and guides the ship by giving form to the movement produced by the much greater but unformed power of its engines.

How does this concept relate to you, your brain, and your behavior? I suggest that it has three important implications. First, as noted previously in discussing the second level of brain neuroplasticity, your primitive Gestalt pattern can be considered the underlying guiding force by which new nerve development takes place.

Then, at the next level of neuroplasticity, when you engage in new ways of thinking, separating yourself from the old primitive Gestalt pattern and switching to a more mature Gestalt pattern, enrichment and changes in your personal social environment will guide brain development along new, more adaptive and resilient patterns.

But the third and most exciting implication has to do with a deeper pattern that I believe Bohm refers to when he talks about the quantum potential. This more subtle force, which permeates the entire universe, is the deepest level of reality. It is variously referred to as "the source," the One, the Life Force. When peak performers tap in to their deepest source of strength and get into the zone, I believe this is what they are getting close to. This can become one of your most powerful resources. It will be discussed further when we look at resilience pillar three, "relationship with something greater."

Let's bring this discussion back to The Path. We can think of your primitive Gestalts as the underlying subtle field or force from which all of your behavior derives. It is the underlying pattern that guides the development of your brain and the process of neurogenesis. This is why, as much as you sometimes struggle to change, you wind up falling back into old patterns. Your primitive Gestalt has a gravitational pull you haven't been able to escape. The new story you just created will help you achieve the third level of neurogenesis. This in turn will encourage new levels of adaptation and resilience. Adhering to this new story will help you stay on The Path.

The ultimate or fourth level of neurogenesis occurs when we source our lives from what Bohm refers to as a deeper, implicate order of unbroken wholeness. Not surprisingly, this is the path and the perspective of many of the ancient traditions. As I guide you onto The Path, we will be working to create a new perspective whose foundation consists of the lessons of today and the reality of who you are today—triggering my third level of neurogenesis. At the same time I will be offering you the opportunity to explore the fourth level of neurogenesis, which can transcend even this optimal place of sourcing and living. Go to step thirteen on The Path now.

STEP 13   *Visualization to trigger neuroplasticity*

The interconnectedness of everything: this will be a visualization designed to stretch your mind a bit further than it has been stretched up to this point.

Doing so will help expand your neurogenesis and gene expression.

Imagine standing on the shore, looking out over a great ocean. Or, alternatively, standing on a high mountain, looking at land stretching to the horizon. In either case, imagine that you are standing with legs relaxed, shoulder-width apart. You begin to deepen your breath and slow it to six breaths per minute (approximately ten seconds for an entire breathing cycle). You survey the view: the sea of water or the sea of land, the horizon, and the endless sky. As you watch the horizon, you can detect its curve—that is part of the curvature of the earth itself. Yes, you can actually detect the curve of the earth, which gives you a sense of the entire planet Earth, as you imagine the curve continuing in both directions. You are sitting on, and are part of, the huge planet Earth. You can see the sun far away in the sky, you imagine the moon somewhere out there and then the planets of the solar system: Mercury, Venus, Mars, Jupiter. All, somewhere out there. Take a moment to imagine—as best as you can—that you are a part of this unfolding universe. Imagine as many parts of this universe as you can wrap your head around. And finally, imagine the implicate order, an invisible force or power underlying everything in your imagination. Feel into the interconnection of everything. Allow its power to enter your body.

USING NEUROPLASTICITY TO ENHANCE YOUR RESILIENCE AND YOUR LEVEL OF SUCCESS

This is your introduction to how we use the concept of neuroplasticity to become more resilient and more capable of achieving higher levels of success. Clearly, as noted, neuroplasticity at levels one and two continue to constrain your learning within old patterns. This minimizes your ability to adapt and bounce forward. It is when you are able to go to levels three and four that you reboot and begin to make breakthroughs in your ability to adapt, adjust, and perform optimally. This is where you find true success.

Any rule that prevents you from fully taking in and utilizing new information interferes with resilience. You are further constrained by inappropriate fears. An easy way to recognize this is by doing steps fourteen and fifteen on The Path now.

STEP 14   *Walking the plank, the easy way*

Imagine a six-inch-wide wooden plank about six feet long on the ground in front of you. Now, imagine walking across this plank. Notice how relaxed you are while doing it and that it presents no difficulty at all.

STEP 15   *Changing perspective changes the experience*

Now that same six-inch-by-six-foot plank is placed across two ten-story buildings, right next to each other. You are standing on the roof in front of the plank and asked to walk across it. Try to really imagine being at that height as you begin to walk across the plank.

You are probably finding it considerably more difficult, if not impossible. (This would certainly be the case if you were actually at that height.) The fear of falling will have an impact on your body and your brain. Your body will tense, making it more difficult to maintain balance. At the same time your brain, fearing for your life, will become less effective and will either freeze or resort to stereotypic and less effective functioning.

Early childhood learning, under the influence of survival instincts, has frozen your abilities, your adaptability, and your resilience—just as it could freeze your movements at the top of those buildings. However, you are now being introduced to The Path and, with each step on The Path, you are breaking free of these old patterns, becoming more resilient, and enhancing your abilities for success.

SIGNPOST

- You have identified a childhood pattern that doesn't serve you.
- You have identified an outmoded message of your internal voice.
- You have listened for the healthy voice, and you have heard it tell you to be more accepting of yourself.
- You have visualized the birthing of your brain cells along new healthy lines of development.
- You have followed through with the visualization of the interconnectedness of everything.

CHAPTER 6

HOW YOU STAND ON THE 9 PILLARS
Your Personal Resilience Profile

et's again define resilience. I have said that resilience is the ability to self-regulate and adapt—so that you can fully and quickly bounce back after any performance or stress. Self-regulation means that when something throws you out of balance, you are readily able to restore that balance. And "out of balance" can be physical, emotional, or mental. If stress or other demands take a lot of energy, you are able to restore those resources rapidly so they are again available for new actions and don't keep wearing you down. This ability also helps you perform better and longer.

"Optimal adaptability" means your ability to make adjustments based on new learning and new experiences about how the world works. In other words, you do not continue with old thinking or behavior that no longer produces the best results, and you don't keep making the same mistakes. Resilience is being aware and awake for as many moments in your life as possible. Each moment that you are awake is a potential moment for enhanced performance. This results in you being more "response-able." Adaptability and new learning require being aware and awake.

In chapter five I explained that resilience includes renewal through the birthing of new nerve cells or brain cells. I then identified four different levels of neurogenesis. Neurogenesis that enhances resilience involves the third and fourth types. This simply means that you are not stuck in your old patterns of childhood lessons and wounding. It is important to be available to integrate new information about yourself and your world. The greater your willingness to challenge existing beliefs, the greater your resilience. This is the source of creativity.

I have also indicated that if you are fearful, your nervous system will be much more active and on guard than that of someone who feels safe. This can be the result of viewing the world as dangerous or unpredictable, or it may reflect your lack of confidence in your ability to handle demands placed on you. In other words, your view of the world and how capable you feel about handling danger are significant factors in your resilience. In fact, we can boil all your efforts down to two categories: defense and growth/repair. When your body is in the defense mode, not only does it put all of its energies into defense, but also this means that other functions, such as maintenance, development, and healing, do not take place. When there isn't a proper balance between these two orientations, when you don't put enough of your body's energies into growth, what happens? Your body begins to break down and not be able to take care of itself.

HEALTH AND HEART RATE COHERENCE

We can make some generalizations regarding resilience. Feelings of love produce more resilience than anger. Anger is appropriate under certain conditions, but being angry or frustrated with the world will leave you less resilient. This has been shown in research looking at heart rate coherence. "Heart rate coherence" refers to the systematic change in your heartbeat from one moment to the next. Although we might give our heart rate a number, say 70 beats per minute, in fact, it's never really a steady 70 beats per minute. Your heart rate is constantly changing, and you can determine the health of your heart by how it changes. First, the greater the range of your heart rate from the fastest beat-to-beat interval to the slowest, the healthier you are. Thus, athletes can have a change in their heart rate of over 40 or 50 beats per minute from fastest to slowest. People with heart disease, on the other hand, have very small changes in heart rate—in other words, very low heart rate variability.

Second, health is a function of the coherence of your heart rate pattern. This is when your heart rate increases in a progressive, orderly manner while you are breathing in, and it decreases in a stepwise fashion as you breathe out.

When you are experiencing feelings of love and gratitude, your heart rate pattern is more likely to be coherent. Conversely, with anger and frustration, there is a disruption of this smooth pattern, and you see more chaotic changes that are less healthy.

Treating yourself with compassion works much better than being self-critical. Many people have developed a pattern of putting themselves down. When I question people about their motivation for doing this, they often say they don't deserve better. But even in cases where people believe they are deserving, they also believe that being hard on themselves motivates them to do better. This may be how your parents trained you, but it is not accurate. Any time you put yourself down, you are giving yourself a mini wound; you are hurting your self-confidence. This can only result in having less trust in yourself and thus making it more difficult for you to succeed. Furthermore, you are negatively affecting your heart rate coherence, which takes a physical toll.

OPTIMAL USE OF PERSONAL OR PSYCHIC ENERGY

Resilience is the optimal functioning of your mind, body, and spirit. It is the optimal use of personal energy, your life force as described in chapter one. Optimal use means using as much as is needed for the task at hand and not an ounce more. In other words, it is the efficient use of your energy. This is in contrast to how most people squander personal energy. For example, my definition of worry is the excessive use of one's resources without any constructive result.

Resilience is also about optimally replenishing the energy used for daily life and peak performance. Many successful people are very good at engaging in hard work to achieve a goal. Resilience, however, includes the ability to replenish your energy after any effort. This involves a conscious process of turning off the activation, releasing the tension of this effort, going inside, and engaging the recuperative process.

Another common waste of personal energy, resulting in less resilience, is your emotional overreaction to people and situations. Your emotional reactions should be in tune with the importance of a situation. Too often, you will react to the unimportant behavior of others—and then feel victimized, blaming others for upsetting you. (We will get into this more in chapter twelve, "Emotional Balance and Mastery.")

Typically, what I'm referring to stems from emotional unfinished business. To achieve high levels of resilience and success, you must be willing to face your demons, face your wounding—emotional experiences that have not been resolved—and go through the healing process. Emotional wounds ignored or suppressed can drain your energy and life force.

With this as introduction, I'd like you to meet my comprehensive nine-component model—the 9 Pillars of Resilience and Success. I've already covered a lot of territory leading up to this point, and you have also taken my Resilience Questionnaire for the first time at the beginning of this book. The good news is that my model incorporates all that is important. It is a systematic approach to personal efficacy and enhanced coping skills for dealing with stress, as well as achieving peak performance along with optimal health. My resilience model incorporates nine components within three unique areas: relationship, organismic balance and mastery, and personal functioning. Following this introduction, you will have an opportunity to retake my Resilience Questionnaire, score your results, and plot these on your second personal Resilience Profile. The result will be a good gauge of where your strengths lie and the areas needing further development. As you compare this profile with the results from your original scores, you may notice some shifting taking place due to your effort and "steps" so far. This is also your starting point as we begin to address the nine pillars.

RELATIONSHIP

Within "relationship," the first area of resilience, there is your relationship with yourself, your relationship with others, and your relationship with something greater. This is about different levels of connection, beginning with your most important connection, the quality of your relationship with yourself.

To whom would you say you are closest? Would it be your partner or spouse, your children, or your parents? Well, there is one person with whom you spend every waking moment of your day and with whom you always go to bed. I'm referring to you. That's right: even though you typically ignore or take this for granted, the person you are closest to and most intimate with is yourself.

How you treat yourself is important because it's a process you engage in twenty-four hours a day, seven days a week. There isn't a moment in which you are not with yourself and very few moments in which you are not, in some way, communicating with yourself. You are the one person you can't hide from.

How well you do in life is so dependent on this relationship. It determines whether you thrive or struggle. So how do you treat yourself? Are you accepting, or do you judge yourself and are frequently critical? Do you give yourself a break, forgiving yourself for your mistakes? Or do you always find something wrong with what you did and continually remind yourself of your errors, perhaps under the misperception that this will push you to do better?

What is your image of yourself deep down inside? Do you harbor feelings of being inadequate and not OK? How do you value yourself? When you do something well, do you give yourself appropriate credit? Do you accept the compliments of others, or do you find a part of what you did that wasn't quite right, feeling as though you should have done better? When you succeed, do you find yourself saying it was just luck, coincidence, or that anybody could have done it, thus minimizing your success? Maybe you feel like you are pulling the wool over people's eyes?

A healthy relationship with yourself that fosters resilience is based on love and acceptance. It facilitates a sense of worthiness and deservedness. This doesn't mean that you are perfect, that you don't hold yourself accountable, or that you don't recognize areas needing growth. It is simply the best approach to personal improvement and self-esteem.

In thinking about your relationship with yourself, we can relate it to how a parent treats his or her child. In a healthy parenting relationship, the intention is to foster growth and good feelings and be loving, supportive, accepting, compassionate, and caring. Of course, part of good parenting is also setting boundaries and sometimes saying, "Yes, I know you want to play, but you have to finish your work first." A good parent doesn't attack, put down, or undermine a child. It simply doesn't work in the long run.

How does your relationship with yourself impact resilience? Well, for starters, whenever you put yourself down, you are impacting your belief in yourself and your sense of worth and competence. Your life feels more uncertain because you feel less capable, so your stress response is triggered more frequently. You also feel less deserving, which makes it more difficult for you to take action or accept success. Research consistently shows that coming from a loving place within yourself triggers healthy heart rate patterns and an internal feeling of harmony, while getting upset with yourself does the opposite, creating physiological disruptions that leave your body feeling tense and impaired.

We can frame this another way. Most people experience them-selves as being in a hole they are trying to climb out of. They see their faults, their inadequacies, and what needs correcting. They are not even at the starting point. This perspective itself is stressful. I suggest that a more effective approach is to believe you are OK and to be accepting of yourself. You are not in a hole. From this place of being OK, you can still identify what needs improvement: "I make mistakes," "I am absent-minded and forget things." But with this latter framework, you will be less stressed, feel more deserving, and achieve greater success.

There is a value without a dollar sign to good relationships, partic-ularly positive, supportive ones. There is value in a friend to whom you can go for an objective appraisal of a situation and feedback that is not colored by jealousy or other conflicting emotions. It is always import-ant to have someone who you know will be supportive and accepting. This second pillar of resilience is your ability to establish and main-tain nurturing and intimate relationships, as well as the ability to make new connections in your personal and professional life. It is also about your effectiveness in choosing the right people—emotionally healthy people—to relate to.

How do your relationships with others translate into greater resil-ience? Let's identify two very different situations in your life. One is with a friend with whom you feel very comfortable, someone you trust and feel is really on your side, wanting you to succeed. Now, think about this person or how you feel anticipating being with them. You probably notice feeling calm, positive anticipation, and a sense of relief. When you are with them, they reflect back to you a sense of being OK.

Now, let's think of another person: Perhaps you feel like you're walking on eggshells around them. Or they may unexpectedly get annoyed or upset with you. Think of how you feel when you are with this person. Notice the difference between these two situations. Uncer-tainty, judgment, and conflict result in the mobilization of your stress response. Too much of this interferes with resilience. Perceiving your environment to be safe allows you to relax. You don't need to be on guard. There is less need for your stress response and physical activation.

The quality of your relationships and your ability to engage with other people can directly impact this dynamic, affecting your level of tension. The more intimate you are able to be with a select group of close friends and relatives, the more positively it will impact your resilience and ability to handle stress and bounce back. Good relationships serve to validate and reinforce a sense of being OK. This affects confidence and a sense of safety, which are key ingredients of resilience.

The third relationship component is your connection with something greater. This can be a spiritual belief or a sense of purpose; it is also a focus on giving service. It is some aspect of yourself that connects you to the larger community or with a spiritual foundation.

Many forces in our modern society cause a sense of isolation that can contribute to depression and despair or simply intensify our experience of stress. Your relationship with something greater allows you to feel more connected and more hopeful. In addition, establishing a longer, bigger horizon for your life smooths out the bumps and curves that are inevitable in daily living. Finally, from a deeper perspective, giving service or giving back to the community fosters a flow of energy. We hear the expressions "what goes around, comes around" and "good karma." They allude to a universal sense of connection where everything is somehow tied to everything else: "When a butterfly flaps its wings in Brazil, it affects the weather in Nebraska." I have noticed for a long time that when I put my energy out—for whatever purpose—something positive comes back to me, although it may come from a totally different direction.

ORGANISMIC BALANCE AND MASTERY

The next area of my resilience model includes the three components of balance and mastery. We need this balance within our physical body, with our thinking or mental patterns, and with our emotions. Let's start with the first: physical balance and mastery. How well are you able to calm down and relax after stressful events or when you need to go to sleep? Can you maintain a sense of calm, or do you find yourself having big reactions to seemingly unimportant situations? Physical balance is about having some control over activating and calming your nervous system.

I see people all the time who come to me because they have low energy, feel drained, or experience constant tension. These are the consequences of triggering your stress response too frequently, too intensely, or for too long, keeping it on long after a stressful situation is over. Most of us have an imbalance between the part of our nervous system that activates to stress and the relaxation component that turns down that activation. Furthermore, we are typically unaware of holding tension in our body.

There is a simple reason for this. We all have countless situations in our lives that trigger the stress response, but how many trigger our relaxation response? Almost none! Furthermore, at times we engage in behaviors that create more stress than is necessary, either to feel more productive or just because we have become accustomed to the feeling that we get with activation.

The next pillar of resilient living is mental balance and mastery. How do you start your day? Are you excited or worried about what the day will bring? When a problem comes up in your life, do you view it with apprehension or as a challenge to be met and overcome? When there is uncertainty, do you have catastrophic expectations, imagining the worst possible outcome? These are examples of your mental orientation to life, your thinking style. A more positive attitude keeps you lifted and embracing life. It actually affects the neurochemistry of your brain, triggering the release of endorphins, the natural chemicals in your brain that help you feel good and even reduce pain. On the other hand, apprehension and focusing on the negative result in overworking your body. This mental orientation leads to a brain with very different biochemical responses, producing a greater sense of anxiety and tension. With these different approaches, two people can go through the same events of the day yet have totally different experiences and feel very different.

Mental balance is also mastery over your thinking and where you place your attention. This means that you can stop thinking about something when you want to. You can turn off the chatter in your head. For example, you can do this in order to fall asleep at night or to focus on a task. You can change the subject of your internal dialogue when you want and not get stuck obsessing about something you have no control over. Sometimes people say to me, "I'm not negative, just realistic." They remind me that even though there's only a 10 percent possibility of a negative outcome, it's still possible and needs to be dealt with. The answer to this is yes: Certainly prepare for possible negative outcomes. But once you plan, dwelling on that potential serves no purpose and leaves you drained, as your body stays tense and on high alert.

The next component of my model of resilience is emotional balance and mastery. You know the expression "someone pushed my button," used to explain why an individual reacted so strongly to a situation. This emotional reactivity is a signal that this person's emotional wounds and/or emotional unfinished business were just activated. This sensitivity impacts resilience in a number of ways. To begin with, when you have such a reaction, you are thrown off balance. Your body activates as with other stresses. It also becomes your focus at the expense of everything else you are doing.

Unfinished business and unresolved feelings engender a propensity for these sensitivities and overreactions. You have more and more buttons that can be pushed, leaving you less and less in control of your life. Instead, you are controlled by all those people and situations that can trigger your emotional reaction.

Your unfinished business doesn't go away on its own. The expression "time heals all wounds" is really not correct. These feelings simply get buried, pushed down, or "depressed" through numbing or other defense mechanisms. You hold in these feelings, leading to physical tension and a reduced ability to experience joy. A part of your psyche is always distracted, trying unconsciously to finish unfinished business. Therefore, addressing these situations enhances your resilience. Any time you are able to get closure, you feel relief and a letting go that allows you to be more present and more capable of addressing the important issues in your life.

Full awareness of one's feelings and the courage to go to difficult emotional places when necessary are the keys to emotional resilience. It is this appropriate experiencing of feelings that allows their release and leaves us available for new possibilities and enhanced personal development.

PERSONAL FUNCTIONING

The last three pillars of resilience and success fall into the category of personal functioning. The first of these is presence. Probably the best way to know what I'm referring to is simply to recall different people in your life and how you feel when you're next to them, as well as the quality of the energy you receive from them. Presence can be divided into two parts: what you project out into the world and how present and aware you are of your external and internal environment, which is the receiving part of presence.

The outward part of presence is the sum total of how you present yourself to the world. Do you project an image of someone who is happy and confident—or somewhat tense and uncomfortable? What is your posture, erect or somewhat bent? What is the expression on your face? Do you look worried and guarded or embracing of the outside world? Are you inviting contact or are you defensive or trying to be invisible?

When you are preoccupied with events of the past or worried about the future, it takes away from your presence. When you are concerned about revealing unwanted parts of yourself, it takes away from your presence. The inward part of presence is how well you are available to receive. It's how well you make contact with the outside world. Are you aware, noticing your surroundings, or are you distracted? Inward presence also includes an awareness of your internal environment.

The next component of your functioning is flexibility. Here are two examples. The first is the willow tree. This tree can withstand strong winds. Its branches bend but don't break. It can withstand tremendous forces because it has flexibility. Another image is from the fable "The Princess and the Pea." It is the story of a princess who was so sensitive she could feel a tiny pea even when it was under twenty mattresses. She was so inflexible that this sensation kept her from being able to sleep. Where do you fall between these two?

Life is complex, and events don't typically all line up the way we would like them to. Flexibility is about being able to take what you can from what is presented and make the best of it, to adjust when your expectations are not met.

The ninth and last component of my resilience model is what I refer to as "power," which I define as the ability to get things done. It's the result of how you interact with your world: how persistent you are, how effective you are, and how focused you are. Power is impacted by your reaction to fear. Does it disable you, or can you summon up courage even if you are afraid? One way you may sabotage your power is by thinking you don't have enough confidence, as if confidence were some innate quality. In fact, confidence is developed on an ongoing basis. Thus, your confidence is enhanced every time you tackle something difficult. Are there some things in your life right now that you are avoiding? Have you been able to identify goals and then go out and reach these goals?

RATING YOUR LEVEL OF RESILIENCE

Let's assess where you are on The Path right now. It is always helpful to have a sense of where you are at points along your journey. Among other things, it will help you recognize your improvement as you follow The Path. In chapter one you completed the Resilience Questionnaire for the first time. Now you can take it for a second time, right before you address the nine pillars but after completing the first six chapters of The Path. The questionnaires and The Path of Resilience Profile can be found on page 373. They can be completed in fewer than ten minutes. When you are finished, you can easily determine your score by adding the numbers for each pillar and getting their totals. Next, go to the second Resilience Profile that follows and plot the totals for each of your pillars in the appropriate location as you did previously. This will give you a personalized profile—your updated Resilience Profile.

As you will notice, different shadings refer to different levels of ability or competency, from low scores (labeled as "problem areas") to "optimal functioning," with in-between levels of "average functioning" and "borderline." This gives you a sense of the areas that need improvement and those you can count on. It might also indicate improvements already achieved as you compare your two completed profiles.

Some people may find many areas that need improvement and few areas of strength. That's OK! This is your starting point as you develop your nine pillars. One of the first lessons is to come from a place of acceptance. This does not mean it's OK to be at this level. It's simply an acknowledgment of what is real, what is true. Right here, right now, this is your level. Until you continue learning the resilience lessons, it is impossible for you to be any place but right here, right now. It is your starting point, but it won't be your ending point. Just remember: any time you get upset by what is, you become less capable of doing the work you need to do to move forward.

At the end of the book, you will have an opportunity to retake both the Resilience Questionnaire and the Symptom Checklist. This will further help you identify your progress and motivate you to continue with The Path, laid out in these chapters.

THE STRUCTURAL SETUP FOR DYSREGULATION

Some of you may be wondering and thinking, "I've done everything I'm supposed to do and followed all the messages from my parents, teachers, and environment. Why am I now struggling? Why is life so difficult?" This is a very good question. If you have been learning the lessons of childhood and life, why are you not doing better and handling stress better?

As I have been indicating, there are structural mismatches that have set you up for becoming out of balance and too stressed. The first mismatch is that your stress response that has evolved over eons is meant for a very different environment than you live in. While your world has advanced into the industrial and information ages, your body is still stuck with the stress-coping response of hunter-gatherers. I'm referring to the fight-or-flight response. Furthermore, trauma can also engage an even more primitive "freeze" response. All this has been discussed previously. Let me ask you: How many of the stresses in your day can be solved by either fighting them or running away from them? The point here is that each time you respond to stress, you push yourself further out of balance, unless you know how to compensate for this mismatch. In particular, your body mobilizes energy for fight or flight, and then you must hold in that energy. That's a big overuse of your precious energy as well as a source of unnecessary tension.

The next problem I've discussed is the developmental mismatch between the environment in which you learned how to use your stress response—your childhood environment—and your current environment. Since you are not able, as a child, to go through your neighborhood (and other neighborhoods) and sample the teachings of many parents and families, you were stuck with the lessons from your environment. And most significantly, the unspoken implication was that the lessons you learned were true for the entire world. And also, that what you learned—including ways that you felt you were not OK—was accurate.

These early lessons, because they are survival lessons and because you are not capable of questioning them, go in very deeply and form the neural networks of your representations of the world and how it works. Again, as suggested by D. O. Hebb: "Neurons that fire together wire together." In other words, you don't question them and feel like they must be true. You then filter messages and lessons from experience that agree with this network and disregard results that don't agree. This is why it is sometimes difficult to take in compliments if it doesn't agree with your narrative.

And the final "nail in the coffin" of dysregulation is the consequence of the learning and conditioning process itself. Think about the successes in your life. I guarantee that most of them were accompanied by stress. Important phone calls, meetings, presentations, or deadlines were all accompanied by stress. In other words, you learned—unconsciously—that stress is associated with success. What do you think this results in? It encourages you to engage in stressful behaviors, expecting they will result in success!

NEED FOR AN ADAPTIVE "REBOOT" TO ESTABLISH DYNAMIC ADAPTIVE BALANCE

As you can see, even if you have learned perfectly and done everything correctly, it has led you down the road to greater and greater dysregulation. Many of the lessons have not served you. Your body is an exquisite instrument. Take a moment and take a few deep breaths, letting the air out slowly. As you do, imagine being a woodwind instrument with the air moving through your body creating the feelings, sounds, and vibrations of your body and your life. But what I'm suggesting is that you have continuously tuned your mind and body to the wrong frequencies, the wrong tuning fork, the wrong lessons!

It is time for an adaptive "reboot." It's time to learn the appropriate lessons and anchor yourself in the most effective ground of life. This new and more accurate center will put you on The Path of success and overcoming the obstacles we all face in our lives. It will lead to your greatest physical, mental, and emotional health. This ground is shared with you over the next nine chapters, in which you will learn the pillars of resilience and success as well as what it takes to be on The Path of optimal functioning.

As noted here, I'm suggesting that this process is no less than the "reboot" of your operating system. It will prompt you to let go of faulty lessons and replace them with lessons that will help you function most efficiently and effectively in your life. This reboot will help you establish an ongoing process I refer to as "dynamic adaptive balance," in which you are available, moment by moment, to appropriately adjust to whatever life throws at you. Return to the Symptom Checklist and Resilience Questionnaire in the appendix on page 373. Observe how your responses may have changed now that you have made it this far in the book.

CHAPTER 7

PILLAR ONE
Relationship with Self

I n over forty years as a therapist, I have marveled at the effort my clients make to change and to grow. These efforts include trying new and difficult behaviors, dealing with their painful emotions, and asserting themselves in their relationships. I see people struggle to free themselves from the controlling influence of a parent or some other toxic relationship. It's as though they are climbing a steep, rocky mountain, achieving one hard-won handhold or foothold at a time.

Yet, so much of the time, an invisible hand seems to reach out to undermine the efforts, digging the dirt and rocks out from under each emotional handhold or foothold, resulting in a backward slide. Despite their battles, clients feel they are not making any progress but instead are going in circles. And despite their achievements, it's difficult for them to take credit and feel good about themselves. What is behind this seeming contradiction? It is their relationship with self!

Everyone, to some degree, fights some form of self-doubt, self-criticism, and the sense of not being OK or enough. These conflicts take you out of alignment and interfere with your purpose and optimal functioning. This makes it difficult to be resilient!

This self-sabotage is typically unconscious as well as unintentional. You may be quick to notice that you need to end a toxic relationship with someone else. But if the problem is how you treat yourself, you are less able to see it or believe it.

YOUR POSITIVE/NEGATIVE SCORECARD

John Gottman, a psychologist at the University of Washington, has determined after thousands of hours of observing couples—both successful and unsuccessful—that in successful relationships, the partners exhibit many more positive behaviors toward each other than negative behaviors. In fact, when the ratio drops below five positive to one negative—a five-to-one ratio—then the relationship is in trouble. And in the most successful and long-term relationships, that ratio is closer to twenty to one! But what about the relationship you have with yourself? How many of you maintain this optimal twenty-to-one, positive-to-negative ratio?

A typical example is Joe, a person who has difficulty meeting people due to social anxiety. In his therapy, when he finally developed the courage to put himself in a social setting, he focused on the negative: what went wrong or what didn't happen. He was self-critical and noted that he shied away from meeting people. In addition, he misinterpreted the actions of others at the gathering, imagining that he was being judged every time someone looked in his direction. (These negative interpretations will be addressed as part of pillar five, thinking and mental balance and mastery, in chapter eleven.)

Joe turned a positive effort—one he should have been proud of accomplishing—into a negative experience. Unfortunately, this was his typical pattern. He would work very hard to accomplish a difficult task and, upon success, he would be relieved and briefly allow himself to acknowledge it. But very quickly after that, he would reflect on something that to his mind wasn't quite right. His critical self would identify how he didn't do it exactly the way it should have been done or that the outcome wasn't exactly as he thought it should be. Before long, all he remembered about the experience was what went wrong.

How does this relate to resilience? Many factors go into how well you bounce forward from the stresses and hassles of your daily challenges, as well as how you achieve optimal performance. In this example, Joe did something that for him was difficult: he attended a social event. Instead of being emotionally nourished by his effort, Joe turned it into a negative. Instead of his effort leading to a gain in confidence, appreciation of his effort, trust in himself, and a reduction in fear surrounding this type of engagement, he stored another negative in his memory banks. That negative interpretation of his experience reinforced his discomfort, leaving him less confident and more fearful about the next time he faced a similar situation.

Unconsciously, Joe may have come to believe that this was the way to get himself to do better, by focusing on what was not done right, what still needed to be done, and the mistakes made—and minimizing the positive aspects of the effort. Or it might stem from a self-directed message of not being OK. Like Joe, many of you are punishing yourselves for mistakes made today, yesterday, or years ago. But any successes you anticipate from this approach are a myth perpetuated by your upbringing. In fact, harping on any mistake only makes its recurrence more likely and perpetuates the sense of being defective and undeserving.

For many, there is no good explanation for why you're hard on yourself and don't give yourself a break. You get angry all too easily—so easily that it's obvious the anger is there all the time, lurking right below the surface, barely hidden. Any little mistake is a good excuse to allow the angry feelings to pour out. When asked about this self-destructive behavior, clients typically say that it somehow "feels" right. In other cases, it appears simply to be what was learned as a child. It's easy to blame yourself for your past mistakes and, sometimes, the mistakes of your family members.

When you are self-critical, you create tension, uncertainty, and low self-esteem—thereby creating more uncertainty about your efforts the next time. In this way, you undermine your success. When you fully accept your positive steps, you provide yourself with a major source of emotional nourishment. It's this nourishment that supports your personal development and self-confidence.

The above examples demonstrate how your relationship with yourself can maintain your fears and lack of confidence. You end up on guard more frequently and find more of your experiences stressful, which triggers your stress response and leaves you more tense and fatigued from day to day.

THE KEY INGREDIENTS FOR A HEALTHY RELATIONSHIP WITH YOURSELF

What are the most important factors in establishing and maintaining a healthy relationship with yourself? We often hear it said that it's impossible to love someone if you don't first love yourself. There is definitely some truth to this statement. In fact, love and acceptance are at the heart of a good relationship with yourself.

Self-acceptance was touched upon in chapter two when we discussed the impossibility of being in two places at the same time. You can't be anywhere other than where you are. If you are someone prone to making errors or not paying attention, then getting angry with yourself and putting yourself down will only cause more distress. You can either accept where you are and relax or you can be upset by it, thus triggering frustration and anger that leave you less able to be fully present (pillar seven), which results in still more errors.

Not long ago, I was trying to untie a knot. When the knot didn't respond to my initial tugging, I got impatient and pulled harder, faster. These efforts only served to entangle the cord more as I became frustrated that it wasn't doing what I wanted. I then put more force into the manipulations. Matters kept getting progressively worse—frustration, anger, tension, more expenditure of energy, more knotting. "Why am I not getting the result I want?" I asked myself. "Why is this cord not cooperating?"

I finally stopped, took a deep breath, sat back, and laughed as I realized what I was so angry about. "Wow, I'm getting angry at a piece of cord, as if this will make a difference." I had to remind myself that this cord wasn't purposely frustrating me by staying tangled. It was simply being a piece of cord.

In this case, as I sat back and looked at the cord, I acknowledged its neutrality and focused specifically on accepting it as it is. I continued to breathe and focused on restoring a sense of calmness. I let go of my anger and antagonistic approach. From that place of calmness, I reengaged the process of untangling the knot. In no time, I was successful! Furthermore, I found that I actually enjoyed the process. Moments like these are simple examples for me to reflect upon the value of acceptance—with myself and with the world around me. (I must also mention that such a big, angry reaction might be a clue that I'm holding in anger from some unfinished business. I will get into this in detail under pillar six.)

Self-acceptance allows for a greater ongoing sense of calmness, which is at the core of resilience. Other components of a good relationship with yourself include being compassionate, giving yourself support, taking good care of yourself, and feeling as though you are deserving. In fact, this means deserving to experience joy and happiness. You want to be able to forgive yourself when you make mistakes, and strive for unconditionally loving yourself. It is also important to be able to take in your achievements and the compliments of others. This is your source of emotional nourishment. In addition, it's important to be willing to set boundaries for yourself and be firm when necessary. This is another part of loving yourself.

INTEGRITY: THE ALIGNMENT OF THE IMAGE YOU PROJECT WITH YOUR BELIEFS ABOUT YOURSELF

It is always in your best interest to create and project out to the world an image of yourself that is most likely to be accepted and rewarded by others. The question rarely asked but of utmost importance is: How well does this image correlate with the person you think you really are and does this image censor aspects of yourself with which you are uncomfortable or even disapproving? This gets to the heart of the first resilience component: your relationship with yourself. The greater the discrepancy between the inner and outer you, the greater your internal conflict and tension, as well as your anxiety over fear of exposure.

For many, the heart of the matter brings a realization that, in some way, you feel defective, flawed, not OK. This sense of yourself typically originates from messages received during childhood. (Even in the most healthy childhood environment, it is difficult to avoid some feelings of inadequacy, as you continually encounter challenges that others, who are more experienced and perhaps bigger or older, are handling better than you are.) These messages then become internalized through the development of your own internal parent. This is a concept first introduced in an earlier chapter with the presentation of primitive Gestalts. You carry this internal parent or voice around with you 24/7, continually reinforcing these negative messages. Many of us run from critical parents only to create our own similar critical voice—except this one we can't run from; it goes wherever we go! As Jon Kabat-Zinn writes, *Wherever You Go, There You Are*. Therefore, you are striving for a positive self-perception that you are happy to project and share with the world.

Unless you have a good relationship with yourself, you will find ways to sabotage or otherwise interfere with your own perception of success. Some of the time this is about whether you feel you deserve good things. An example is John, another former client. Although he had a good job, worked hard, and was valuable to his company, he was always second-guessing himself and would dwell on what he did or might have done wrong. In his relationships, he would wonder if the other person really enjoyed being with him.

What is interesting about John is that he consistently received positive feedback. Whether at work or with friends or acquaintances, the majority of what he heard was positive; he did a good job, and people liked him. Exploring his anxieties, it became clear that he always found some way of dismissing the compliments and excellent job evaluations. He would say, "Yes, but . . ." and follow this with what he thought he was not doing well. At work, a good evaluation would be followed by fears of not being able to keep living up to the positive reviews.

Sometimes there are good intentions in being self-critical. On the surface it might seem that you are being critical in order to coerce self-improvement by trying harder. Instead, it keeps reminding you that you're not good enough, that there is something wrong with you, or that you're lazy. This, in turn, undermines your confidence and your trust in yourself that you can do something well. This can only interfere with taking positive actions in your life.

Some clients would ask, "Well, then, what should I do when I so totally blow it and disappoint myself, when I forget something important, when I do something so stupid that a six-year-old would have done it better?" Right, and everyone has those experiences.

What you need to ask yourself is: "What's my goal?" If your goal is to do better the next time, if it is to learn from your mistakes, then it's important to be compassionate and forgive yourself. This is supremely important, as it is apparent that people continue to hold themselves accountable for performing poorly in their childhood, such as getting bad grades in school. Ask yourself, "How long must I suffer for those mistakes?" In fact, your suffering should be met by a supportive and compassionate posture toward yourself.

In 1991, Terry Anderson, a US journalist, was released by the Hezbollah after being held hostage in Lebanon. Anderson was held for 2,454 days! It was the longest confinement suffered by any hostage. In an interview shortly after his release, he was asked if he was plagued by the memories of his ordeal. His response was so profound I remember it to this day. Anderson said, "I went through a terrible and painful 2,454 days; why would I make it worse by continuing to think about it?" When you are suffering due to the consequences of a mistake, ask yourself a similar question: "I am upset because my mistake led to painful consequences. If they are so unpleasant, why make them worse now by holding on to these memories and engaging in self-punishment?"

This brings you to this chapter's first process on The Path—addressing mistakes and bad decisions. Holding on to your past mistakes is a drag on your progress. It is time to release the parts of the past that hold you back—to stop fretting over mistakes. It is the beginning of the process to forgive yourself so you can give yourself a clean slate, a fresh start, and let go of excess baggage. The following process can be used whenever you find yourself angry or are putting yourself down for a mistake or a regret. I suggest you identify something you have been upset at yourself about and follow the lessons below.

PROCESS TO RELEASE EMOTIONAL ENERGY MOBILIZED BY A MISTAKE

So, for example, what do you do about your anger, the anger you have toward yourself that accompanies a mistake? The answer? It is OK to express anger toward yourself at times, but you must abide by certain rules. First, restrict that anger to the specific mistake, for the specific behavior—and don't put yourself down, be self-abusive, or otherwise undermine yourself. (This may sound trivial, but every time you call yourself "a jerk," for example, these words unconsciously sink into your brain.)

Keep the expression of anger in proportion to the situation and give it a time limit. That's right; give yourself, say, five minutes to express the anger. Check the clock.

At the end of the time period, take the next step, which is finding the lesson to learn from the mistake. If you made a mistake, you did something that had a "cost" to you. For the sake of balance, and to feel that there was some "value" to the cost, you must find something you learned from the experience. In other words, the lesson gives value to the experience, making acceptance of the mistake and letting go easier. It also makes it less likely that you will make the same mistake again.

Yes, the last step in this process is to let go of the mistake so you don't, in some way, carry it around, which distracts you from being present and makes you feel less worthy. The way you let go of a mistake is by acknowledging that you have paid a price—the cost of the mistake and the expression of anger toward yourself—and that you have actually learned something from the error. This, in turn, gives the mistake some value. Finally, in a heart-to-heart talk with yourself, recognize that if you love yourself and really want the best for you, you have to show some self-compassion. You have already paid a price for the mistake; letting go is the right way to recover. This leaves you more in the present and, thus, more likely to get it right the next time.

If you are not used to treating yourself this way, you might find it difficult to do it effectively at first. Keep in mind that this is a learning process. You have old patterns that are built into your brain circuits. They are your default mode or automatic response. But each time you follow this process, you are literally creating new nerve circuits or, as Donald Hebb called them, "cell assemblies" that reinforce this process and help make it easier. Go over to The Path, identify one of your mistakes that you still carry around, and go through the process of "addressing mistakes."

STEP 1 *Addressing Mistakes*

If you blow it, make a poor decision, or otherwise do something that sets you back, it can quite naturally cause you to be angry with yourself and to keep going over your mistake and its consequences.

OK, so you made a mistake and are angry with yourself. Here is a six-part process to address your feelings and let go of the mistake.

Identify either a current or past mistake to use and apply the following process:

1. Notice and accept the feeling, but connect the feeling to the behavior and not to who you are! In other words, "I'm angry at myself for locking the keys in my house," rather than, "Wow, I'm really stupid for locking the keys in my house."

2. Allow yourself to express this anger, but give yourself a time limit, say, five minutes. Express your feelings in any way that feels right: write them down, punch a pillow, yell, or scream. Remember, the purpose is to get your feelings out (this is what is unfinished and needs to be expressed in order to let go), not to change events or another person.

3. Be compassionate with yourself. If you did something that will cost you, and you are upset that it cost you, you don't want to add to that cost by beating yourself up. Instead, have compassion for what you are going through. And you also want to have compassion for yourself if you are someone who has difficulty staying focused and thus are prone to mistakes. This is part of loving yourself.

4. What is the lesson to be learned? If you just did something that cost you, you need to find a benefit to attach to this cost. When you find the lesson to be learned, you'll be less likely to make the same mistake in the future.

    If you keep forgetting your keys, make the decision to create some kind of reminder or place an extra set of keys outside your house. Take some action to ensure a better outcome the next time.

5. Accept what has happened. Acceptance doesn't mean you like what happened. It just means that you are accepting reality, that the past can't be changed; it is what it is. You are accepting your actions or inactions that led to the mistake, and you are accepting that this is where you are on your path at this

moment. You are still a person who makes these kinds of mistakes. However, this acceptance leads to . . .

6. Forgiveness and letting go. Finally, it is time to forgive yourself and let go of any resentments. This is the healthy approach and leaves you feeling stronger.

It also leaves you more capable of being in the moment and not distracted by unproductive thoughts. The result is a greater likelihood of improved future performance.

HOW NEGATIVE SELF-TALK AFFECTS YOU—DON'T MAKE WAR ON YOURSELF!

I refer to negative self-talk as self-abuse. This means to treat yourself in a harmful, injurious, or offensive way. So, let's look at the consequences of this negative self-talk or ongoing self-criticism. The most obvious is the hurt. It's an emotional hurt whenever you put yourself down. Typically, the way you deal with this hurt is to somehow become numb, distracted, or otherwise unconscious so you don't notice the emotional pain. None of this is good for awareness, energy, or the ability to feel joy. It causes physiological damage as well. Research has demonstrated that negative emotions can affect how your heart and your brain function.

Next, this approach undermines your self-efficacy—your belief in yourself—resulting in self-doubt. This only makes future actions more difficult and adds to your stress. It also fosters anxiety and worry as you wonder if someone else will discover your shortcomings. You're waiting for the other shoe to drop.

The process of change or personal development always begins with an increased awareness, a noticing. Most of how you behave—whether it's your internal mental thoughts or your external actions—is based upon your habit patterns. By definition, habits are performed outside of your awareness; they are automatic. As such, they are inaccessible. Even when you tackle something new, you typically approach it in the same familiar way you approach everything else.

When you look at your overall habit patterns, they include certain categories. Among them: how you talk to yourself and treat yourself, as well as what you expect from others and from the world. Is your orientation one in which you are expecting others to be hostile or friendly? The summation of these habit patterns is what I have been referring to as your primitive Gestalt.

As noted previously, these patterns were learned in reaction to your childhood environment. And while they served you and were appropriate to get you through your early years, they were specific to who you were then and what you had to deal with at that time in your life. In other words, we can say that you learned these lessons very well. In fact, you were smart. But these lessons you learned so well no longer serve you. It is now up to you to observe and review these patterns, as objectively as possible, with the goal of learning new and more effective approaches to treat yourself and operate in today's world.

Fritz Perls said it this way: "When you are a child you swallow everything whole. Now it's time to chew on these lessons and decide which taste right and you want to swallow and properly digest, and which you want to spit out."

Right now I would like you to become more aware of a key aspect of your primitive Gestalt: how you talk to yourself and how you treat yourself. The first step in the process of addressing old patterns or habits is to become more and more aware of the pattern and when it is occurring. It's about making the unconscious conscious. To do this, go to step two on The Path now to "stalk your pattern."

STEP 2 *Stalking your pattern and your internal voice*

This involves observing—or stalking—how you treat yourself and how your internal voice talks to you.

One way of doing this would be to notice whether you are giving yourself more positive messages than negative ones. More accepting or more critical messages? See how close you come to the twenty-to-one ratio that determines a good relationship with yourself.

Carry a small pad and pen with you throughout your day as an awareness tool. Use it to keep track of your positive and negative internal dialogue.

Visualize an animal stalking its prey, say a large cat such as a jaguar. Notice how focused it is when observing its prey. Try to approach your task with the same level of intensity. Find a way to remind yourself to observe, such as linking this process with important moments in your day. At the end of the day, take a moment to reflect and review the entries on your pad to see how you treated yourself this day. Notice if the process itself, of stalking your pattern, changes your behavior.

COMPARING YOUR INTERNAL VOICE WITH THAT OF A HEALTHY INTERNAL VOICE OR PARENT: CHECKING YOUR "SIGHTS" (FOR ACCURACY)

In this step of the process, note that your "sights" might be off. Here the analogy is to a sharpshooter. If an expert shooter fires at a target and the bullet hits a foot to the left of the target, it would be surprising. He or she would try again, making sure to follow long-standing procedures to do better and hit the target. If the bullet hits a foot to the left again, the shooter will begin to suspect something is wrong. After the third time with the same results, it will be obvious that there is something off with the sighting device or some other defect in the gun.

In understanding your process, it's important to consider that your "sights," your basic self-checking or filtering mechanism, might likewise be a bit off. But here, you can't simply check for a mechanical problem. Instead, use the guides that have been created in The

Path to give you new "sights" and direction. Go to step three on The Path now.

STEP 3　*Comparing with a healthy parent*

This step isn't about trying to change your internal voice but simply to notice how this voice compares to the qualities of a healthy and more effective internal voice. It's a process of "objective noticing," or at least as objective as you can be.

Your "sights" might be off! The lens through which you view yourself and the world may be clouded by your history. The place you go to inside to get a feeling for something might not be accurate—even though it's very familiar. There are some true standards for whether your internal voice—internal parent—is accurate.

Healthy parents want good things for their child and are forgiving of mistakes.

A healthy parent comes from a place of:

- love,
- acceptance,
- support,
- caring,
- compassion, and
- a desire for joy and happiness

while setting boundaries and holding you accountable.

"Setting boundaries and setting responsibilities" guard against your laziness and ensure accountability and progress on The Path.

The next step is comparing the voice you are stalking—your internal voice, the voice of your primitive Gestalt—with the qualities of a healthy internal parent.

These healthy qualities should be considered the more accurate and optimal "sights" or guiding principles.

OBJECTIVE NOTICING

How is it possible to be objective when you are observing yourself? Let's do what I'll call a "thought experiment." A thought experiment is when you imagine conditions or experiences that are not immediately doable. Physicists, such as Albert Einstein, engage in thought experiments to visualize mental scenarios that cannot actually be created in order to work out their theories.

Your thought experiment is to think of someone in your life whom you dearly love. It might be one of your children or a close friend. It can't be someone with whom you are in competition or jealous of. It must be someone you truly desire to be happy; you want that person to have everything he or she wants in life. Usually this is your child or your closest friend. With this person in mind, go to step four on The Path and engage in the described thought experiment.

STEP 4 *Thought experiment*

I'd like you to think of something you did that you continue to be upset about and are having difficulty letting go of. It might be a recent experience or something from a long time ago. It might be a performance you gave that you have judged to be bad, and you're still upset with yourself over it. It's a regret, or something that you continue to be annoyed about or that you use to put yourself down.

Now I'd like you to imagine that it was your child or your close friend who did this—not you. And he or she came to you upset about what he or she did. How will you respond?

In most cases, you will not see it in as negative a light as you see your own behavior. Most likely, you will encourage your friend or child to be forgiving of himself or herself. You would put this experience in a larger context of other behaviors in which this person generally did well. You'd find more positive ways of viewing this situation. And you'd probably say, "Don't be so hard on yourself."

Now, simply take a moment to sit with the difference in how you just treated this other person in comparison to how you treat yourself over the same situation. Is there any legitimate reason why there should be a difference? The answer is no.

YOUR INNER VOICE IS NOT PART OF YOUR GENETIC MAKEUP

There will be a problem believing this at first. The voice you notice is a major part of your primitive Gestalt pattern. Because this voice is embedded in who you are, it is difficult to be objective and clearly recognize its inaccuracies. Since this voice began to develop during the earliest years of your life as an element of your survival mechanism, it has become a part of you and is familiar and comfortable; thus you have difficulty recognizing its destructive qualities.

To help you gain some perspective, it's important to begin thinking of this voice as something that developed after you were born. It is not a genetic part of you that can't be separated out. In other words, it's an "add-on" and not found in your genetic makeup. Go to step five on The Path now to visualize this inner voice as an add-on.

STEP 5   *Considering your existing inner voice as an "add-on"*

Take a moment right now to put everything aside. Get comfortable, breathe easily, four seconds in and six seconds out, letting go of any muscle tension and also letting go of any business in your head.

Visualize yourself as a tiny infant, just coming into the world. Make the connection with this innocent and beautiful little person as being the earliest manifestation of your spirit and the union of your parents' genetic makeup.

Visualize that this little person is still a blank slate waiting to develop based upon learning experiences yet to come.

Most important, visualize this baby that is you waiting to learn how to think, how to feel, and how to be. He or she has yet to establish criteria for this and has yet to develop an internal voice! In other words, that voice is an "add-on," something yet to be learned.

Now, visualize connecting with this beautiful infant; appreciate him or her with all the promise of the future and give him or her new internal messages.

Messages of a healthy internal voice (say this to that baby):

"No matter what, I love you."

"You are a good soul."

"You deserve to have good things in your life and for good things to happen to you."

"There may be things you still need to learn and ways of improving. You may be prone to making mistakes and not paying attention, but remember one very important message: You are OK."

A HEALTHY INTERNAL VOICE

Getting on The Path will frequently require ignoring or saying no to the messages coming from your inner pattern or inner voice. You will have great resistance to letting go of something that has been with you for your entire life. You will struggle to say no to that voice unless you have a second voice: a new, healthier voice to which you can turn. You facilitate your ability to say no when you become aware of an alternative voice.

It's like asking someone to let go of a lifeline without the availability or presence of another source of safety; thus, it's important to develop an alternative voice to call on and listen to.

In chapter two, the concept of your inner voice was introduced, along with how you talk to yourself. You were guided through a dialogue between your existing inner voice and a new voice you want to encourage and develop. This latter voice is associated with the part of you that wants to be healthy and function optimally. It's the part of you that decided to read this book and commit to The Path. As noted, your existing inner voice can be considered the spokesperson for your primitive Gestalt. But more than just a spokesperson, it is also the defender or upholder of the old pattern. It is entrusted with maintaining the status quo.

Why maintain the old pattern if it no longer serves you? The reasons are many, and an understanding of your internal psychological perspective is very important if you are going to break free of it. Remember, your earliest learning was in the service of survival, the most primitive instinct of all. Mother Nature doesn't fool with survival. Nothing else matters if you don't continue to live. Early learning therefore becomes locked into the most primitive survival mechanisms of the brain.

They then become self-maintaining due to their association with survival. It is through these mechanisms that self-criticism and other less than optimal patterns encountered during early years get linked with staying safe. Even though they are not the reasons for your survival, they can be mistaken for necessary ingredients in life.

Let's approach this issue from a different direction. Faced with the fact that they are getting in their own way and negating their best efforts, most people are incredulous. It's very difficult to see it. What I typically hear is, "I'm just being realistic." Or sometimes my supportive comments will be dismissed as coming from someone being paid to be nice.

The true fact is that there is the "Trojan horse" effect. The ancient Greek story goes that after a fruitless, ten-year siege of Troy, the Greeks built a huge horse within which a select force of about thirty men hid.

The Greeks pretended to sail away, and the Trojans pulled the horse into their city as a victory trophy. That night the Greek force crept out of the horse and opened the gates for the rest of the army, which had sailed back under cover of night. The Greek army entered and destroyed the city of Troy.

As the Trojans unwittingly invited the Greeks into their city, as a child you unknowingly let in a voice that took hold inside your psyche. You see, during the developmental process, one of the ways you are able to separate from your caregivers is to internalize aspects of them that you can carry with you. Sometimes it is their actual mannerisms or their coping style that you develop through the modeling process. If the caregivers are critical of you, that criticalness becomes part of your own pattern. If they are always looking for what might be wrong or expecting something bad to happen, this perspective tends to become part of your internal voice. Sometimes messages from teachers and other authority figures reinforce this process.

How you treat yourself is a function of the way you talk to yourself. Everyone has an internal voice. As you grow up and separate developmentally from your parents, you automatically internalize aspects of their teachings and their view of the world along with the messages of society. You incorporate this into your own internal parent, that voice that is always with you. Your internal parent may make unreasonable demands, point out what you did wrong, and keep you on edge. Or it might simply be trying to keep you safe by keeping you within "safe" behavioral boundaries. The irony is that you unconsciously believe you need this voice, this "internal parent," and that without it you would be lost or perhaps make wrong decisions. An important part of developing resilience is the realization that this voice itself is what keeps you stuck, and resistant to new approaches.

Another way of looking at this voice is to realize that as children, we take in everything, unfiltered, without the ability to critically evaluate. As mentioned previously, we swallow these messages whole (like the Trojan horse)—without chewing on them. Part of your process now will be to notice the messages of this voice, to chew on them and determine whether they taste right. Those messages that "taste right"—that are healthy and supportive—you can take back in or swallow as part of yourself. Those messages that don't "taste right" once you chew on them—that are harmful, self-abusive, etc.—you can now choose to spit out.

WHAT "FEELS RIGHT"

One result of this voice being with you your entire life is that what "feels right" will be in alignment with your old pattern and your existing internal voice. Unfortunately, the very place you typically tune in to determine what feels right and what feels wrong—what decision to make, what action to take, and what to believe—is your existing primitive Gestalt and its inner spokesperson.

Remember the analogy I gave you of an expert sharpshooter? In this case, you're the sharpshooter. You aim your gun at the target, shoot, then observe a hole six inches to the left of the center of the target. You pick up the gun again, aim—this time very carefully—shoot . . . and again notice that the bullet hit the target in exactly the same location, six inches to the left. In fact, each time you aim and shoot, you hit the target in the same spot. It's time to tell yourself, "My aim is off," or, more precisely, "My thinking—and what feels right—is inaccurate."

I know it will be hard for you to question your personal "sights." Again, this is because they were established as part of your survival learning as a child. In fact, primitive Gestalts have a neuroanatomical and neurobiological representation. Your brain has formed based upon your primitive Gestalts. They have become imprinted in your brain's cell assemblies. Go to step six on The Path, right now, to engage in a process to address what feels right.

STEP 6 *What feels right?*

Refer back to a mistake of yours or a performance you are still upset about. It might feel right to keep putting yourself down for this, thus reinforcing that you are not OK.

Reflect on how this event has caused you to hurt yourself emotionally. In other words, if you have been angry with yourself, if you have not been able to let go of your criticalness, you must be experiencing an emotional hurt—caused by your own reaction. True, the mistake itself might have resulted in some pain, but continuing to carry it with you has hurt you more deeply. You are extending the negativity of the experience.

As part of your responsibility to love yourself, it is important to be able to console yourself under any form of duress. This needs to trump any urge to put yourself down. So, right now, please review how both the event and your reaction to it have been a source of emotional pain.

Take one of your hands and gently caress your other hand while expressing your sadness at your own suffering. This isn't about right or wrong, good or bad. With this example we want to begin a process of adjusting "what feels right." Ultimately what feels right is loving, accepting, and having compassion for yourself. Continue to caress your hand and give yourself new and more loving messages, such as, "I'm sorry you are in this pain." And, "Remember, no matter what mistake you make, I will always love you."

ACCEPTANCE AND TAKING IN YOUR SUCCESSES AND STRONG EFFORTS

A most important part of your relationship with yourself is fully accepting and appreciating yourself, the positive moves you make, and your successes along the way—and not doing anything to undermine these successes. In fact, sometimes it is simply about appreciating your hard work and effort, no matter the material results.

Think of climbing a mountain. Moment by moment you are trying to find the best handholds and footholds. You struggle and reach, and your hand finds a good hold. To secure this new and advanced position, you would hammer in a piton and secure your rope through it.

Now you have locked in your effort and your new advanced position. Even if you make a misstep that leads to a fall, you will be caught and saved by this newly established position. What you should not do is then use your hands to dig the dirt or rocks out from under this new, secure position, eroding your forward progress. So you shouldn't do this in your life either, and that means fully owning—or accepting—your successes.

Many of my clients have difficulty acknowledging their successes and owning the abilities that helped achieve those successes. When we delve into their resistance, it typically centers on the fear of becoming too cocky. In this approach we are not talking about bragging or puffing out your chest without any support to back you up. This is simply about speaking or thinking the truth, your truth about yourself. This is what establishes self-support and self-confidence.

For many years I took pride in my facility to master geometry in high school. I was able to work through the proofs in many cases without using the textbook. Whenever I had self-doubts, this experience gave me confidence and served as an anchor for my abilities. I could always point to that class to appreciate my gifts and give me confidence in my current activities.

What can you point to? Do you have an academic or athletic success on which you can focus as a reminder of your ability to master a subject or an activity? Perhaps it's a good business deal or doing a good job being a mother or father. Use this to push aside self-doubt and to renew a confidence that serves as an anchor for your abilities. Point to it and remind yourself to appreciate that gift for a boost to your self-esteem.

How many of your past successes have you fully appreciated? Have you fully acknowledged these positive experiences? When you are able to do this and integrate these experiences, there is an unconscious "knowing" of your abilities and your capabilities. This increases your capacity, like having a bigger engine that drives you.

Right now, go to steps seven and eight on The Path and accept some of the good qualities and abilities you have demonstrated through some of your activities. It might be something you did today or it could be from many years ago.

STEP 7 *Strengthening your relationship with yourself; owning your successes*

Identify something you have done really well—something you worked hard to achieve. It might even be surviving a childhood that was particularly difficult.

Review this experience and identify what abilities or skills you needed and demonstrated for this accomplishment.

Write down these special abilities or skills. Take a moment to "take in" or accept these abilities.

Breathe deeply: breathe in the success and your gifts, and as you exhale, imagine projecting these gifts out into the world.

Affirmation: "I trust and have confidence in my abilities."

"I accept myself and my uniqueness."

"I truly and deeply want good things to happen for me."

At the end of each day, sit with your journal for The Path. Simply review your day and take note of the effort you made to create a day of success. In addition, take note of any successes you had. Write these down in your notebook and take a moment to appreciate your effort, your successes, and the abilities they demonstrate. Repeat these affirmations as needed.

STEP 8 *Taking in more of your hard work*

Don't stop now. Give yourself another moment to identify other areas of your hard work. Appreciate first the effort you made for improvement of yourself or of others. Next, identify what positive aspects of yourself and your abilities these efforts demonstrated. For a few moments, simply breathe and allow yourself to feel good about yourself.

Related to this is your ability to take in compliments as well as your successes, which I refer to as "emotional nourishment." This is important, as it helps you to feel OK and not have to continually produce in order to be OK. This makes it easier for you to take time for yourself, to restore yourself, and to be more resilient.

It is also the process by which you open to yourself. When you "accept" or receive appropriately, you let down your guard, your defenses. You are opening in to yourself. At these moments, you may even notice tears in your eyes. You may have experienced this in the past when you unexpectedly began to cry but weren't feeling sad. It may occur in a beautiful moment, or when hearing accolades heaped on a public figure, or while watching a poignant moment in a movie. I refer to this as "melting" and letting go. How resilient you are is facilitated by this process of opening and connecting to emotional places deeper inside yourself. Do step nine now.

STEP 9   *Emotional nourishment—accepting the love and appreciation of others.*

Here I'm using the word "accepting" to indicate taking in and appreciating compliments, love, and support of others. This is as important—perhaps more important for your well-being—as food.

We will do this process in two stages: within your social world of friends and family and then in your business and career world.

Identify one or two people in your family or circle of friends who have, from time to time, given you compliments or in some way have indicated that they admire you or admire what you do.

Take a moment to review these compliments in their entirety. Hear them all over again, while picturing the person or people who said them. Breathe, and as you inhale, allow yourself to fully take in and own these statements—without any qualifications or "buts."

Imagine opening yourself emotionally in order to take them in as deeply as possible. Imagine that by doing this you are receiving emotional nourishment that further supports self-acceptance and your development of resilience.

Next, review your business career. Identify any successes you have had and take a few minutes to appreciate and accept them as well.

Ultimately, resilience—which means your ability to restore, replenish, regenerate, and grow—is about your connection to your "source," your deepest psychic place. When you open and take in positive feedback, you are gaining greater access to this source.

When you have a good relationship with yourself, it means you trust and have confidence in yourself, and you accept yourself with all your blemishes. Now you truly and deeply want good things to happen for you. It results in your personal integrity, the most harmonious relationship between your internal and external worlds. It allows for your physical, mental, and emotional selves to operate at their highest levels.

In working with athletes to achieve peak performance, the concept of calm focus has a huge application. One of the greatest challenges for athletic success is performing under pressure, when it really counts, when everything is on the line. The athlete who can connect with his or her deepest internal source has fewer doubts and worries less about the opinions of others or the outcome. This is a key to peak performance as well as resilience.

FURTHERING YOUR INTERNAL DIALOGUE

Return now to the internal dialogue begun in chapter two between your primitive Gestalt voice and the nascent voice of a healthy, wise parent. Remember how your internal voice, your reference point, can get off track in its service to you, and how you can develop an inappropriate and self-defeating internal voice and self-concept.

If you had a parent who was cold, depressed, or distracted by personal worries and thus unable to be present or nurturing, you would not—as a young child—be able to be objective, to reason: "I know my mother had a difficult childhood and she can't do any better." Instead, your unconscious conclusion would be that "there must be something wrong with me." You see, to recognize your parent's inability to be nurturing or loving would jeopardize your hope of ever getting your emotional needs met. By blaming yourself, and making it your responsibility, at least there is a chance that if you keep trying, you might get it "right," and your parent will respond.

You might wonder what you did to cause your parents to withhold their love. You might have decided—unconsciously—you were not good enough, so you kept trying harder. When nothing worked, the next step was to try to be perfect in order for them to show their love. Of course, you're typically not aware of this process.

As you can see, this can lead to all sorts of inappropriate messages that you give yourself. These messages find their home in an internal parent that is critical, judgmental, or unaccepting. It also results in your inexhaustible efforts as you continually try to do more or always be productive—still trying to fill that emotional void inside.

You might notice that even when you achieve success, the good feelings don't last. Of course, no matter how much you do or get, it will never substitute for this emotional need; it's a dead-end street!

In chapter twelve, "Emotional Balance and Mastery," you will have an opportunity to engage in a process to address some of the wounding and unmet needs of your childhood. In the meantime, this next step on your path will continue the exploration of your existing internal voice and the messages you give yourself. Go to step ten on The Path now to engage in the next dialogue.

STEP 10   *Engaging your internal dialogue at a point where you're stuck*

1. Identify a personal point where you're stuck or in conflict. This might be in your career or a relationship.
2. Engage in a dialogue between the two voices as outlined. Use two chairs so that each voice has its own physical location. This will help you foster the distinction between the voices.

Begin to notice the qualities of each voice. Even though the old voice might sound accurate and correct, that isn't the issue.

Notice whether the voice is focusing on aspects of yourself or your behavior that are undermining, negative, or punitive.

When you shift into the new, healthier internal voice, the keys would be: positive, constructive, compassionate, and optimistic.

You might also note that on this side you are experiencing some annoyance with the negative or critical voice. This is OK. It's OK to be angry and even to express this feeling within the dialogue. Here you are learning to be assertive in the service of meeting your needs and standing up for yourself.

Be careful not to fall into the trap of the old voice's logic. This dialogue isn't about right or wrong. You don't want to simply be right about how you make mistakes or how you are incompetent or ineffective.

These negative messages simply perpetuate self-defeating approaches.

Give yourself an adequate number of times that you switch between the two sides. Always give the new and healthy voice the last word.

SHIFTING POWER AND YOUR "CENTER OF GRAVITY" FROM THE OLD TO THE NEW INTERNAL VOICE

As you begin exploring your primitive Gestalt patterns and their spokesperson, the old internal voice, it will be quite evident that it holds the power, that it is dominant. It typically doesn't allow any other opinion or position. You might say that you have totally identified with that voice. Fritz Perls, one of the founders of Gestalt therapy, referred to this aspect of yourself as your "top dog." This dominance prevents any other internal voice from being heard.

When you are "of two minds," as the expression goes, two different opinions fight it out within you. The Gestalt process you are learning is helpful because it externalizes this fight through the use of the empty chair. This allows the softer "seedling" its chance to speak. It gives the less-developed and less-supported voice—i.e., the newer and healthier internal parent—an opportunity to be heard. It also begins the process of constructively countering the arguments and rationale presented by the old internal voice.

Let me give you an example: You might want to achieve a goal in business and begin planning the first step. Two weeks later, you realize you haven't accomplished anything. "Why am I procrastinating?" you ask yourself. Here is what the ensuing dialogue might sound like.

In one chair, you put the part of you wanting to achieve success. This part might say: "I want to achieve this goal; I want to be successful." You would then switch chairs and have your old internal voice respond.

It might say: "Yes, get on it, get moving; but remember that the last time you tried, you made all kinds of mistakes. You'd better be careful. You don't want to say the wrong thing, as you usually do, and have people think you're stupid." Now you begin to realize why you have been procrastinating! You may believe the voice of the negative internal parent is helpful, but it actually undermines you.

So, as you switch chairs again, your intention needs to be the creation and amplification of a place inside you that is more positive and supportive. While you might already have a sense of this internal voice, consider modeling this voice based on how a good, healthy parent might talk. That model might be someone you know, or it might be a character in literature or the movies, anyone who demonstrates the following qualities: loving and compassionate, accepting, supportive and encouraging, and never abusive. You want your internal voice to be nurturing, while also being firm, protective, and able to set boundaries.

So, as you switch chairs again, this new or strengthened wise internal voice needs to do two things: come from a more positive place and, at the same time, not allow the other voice to be abusive. It might therefore respond: "I don't want you to keep mentioning my mistakes— unless it is to learn from them." Right now, go to step eleven on The Path to continue your dialogue process.

STEP 11 *Shifting your center of gravity to your new voice*

Identify a way that you can be hard on yourself, such as focusing on what you got wrong instead of what you got right. You might acknowledge success, then quickly add a "but." You might expect to make a mistake or you might make some other negative comment about yourself.

In the other chair, give your newer, more positive voice the opportunity to respond. Allow this voice to be more assertive and set a boundary such as, "It's not OK to put me down." Or, "If you can't say anything nice, don't say anything."

I don't expect this positive side to have all the answers or even be able to silence the critical voice. Remember, this is a learning process that will take time. What I'd like you to do is reach deeper inside yourself to find your inner strength. The goal is to be able to simply say something like this:

"I will keep speaking up, even if I don't silence you. I will label you inappropriate and not listen to you even if you speak. I'm not going to give up until the center of gravity shifts from your side to my side."

When you are able to connect deeply—to be able to say with conviction that you are not going to give up—the other side of you will be on the run!

Remember the two lessons about how your brain operates: (1) it wants to hold on to the status quo, and (2) it has a great capacity for "neuroplasticity," the growth of new nerve cells and new nerve pathways. Left to its own devices, it will go with number one. But with intention and by maintaining focus on The Path, your brain will—step-by-step—gradually trigger the growth of new nerve cells and then new nerve pathways that support the healthier behavior and the healthier internal voice. Right now go again to The Path and do steps twelve and thirteen to address the old voice that won't be quiet.

STEP 12   *Continuing to strengthen your new voice*

Think again of a place where you've gotten stuck or are being hard on yourself. You can continue with the example you have already used or choose a new one. Get into a dialogue between the part that is getting you stuck and the new internal voice.

For some of you, the new voice might be timid or difficult to iden-tify, but it is there, somewhere. However small it is, allow it to respond. Its existence is very important.

And remember, this is a learning process. Continue the dialogue as a way of gaining awareness of how you treat yourself, as well as to begin nurturing this more healthy and positive internal voice or parent.

STEP 13   *Hearing but not listening or reacting*

Some of you may get stuck because you just can't stop the old voice, and you believe that the only success is when you silence this voice. The good news is that you don't have to stop the voice in order not to listen to it.

The first stage in shifting from the old negative or critical voice to a new healthy internal parent is simply to hear it and know that it is an old and inaccurate message that no longer serves you.

Noticing without reacting is very powerful. It is an aspect of mind-fulness. The more you can hear the old voice and label it for what it is—outdated and not helpful—the happier and more successful you will be. Use this, or a similar expression, to label the old voice whenever you hear it.

STEP 14   *Taking time for self-care*

Self-care includes taking time to exercise, eat well, get sufficient sleep, and relax. This is all part of developing resilience. Please do the following:

1. Take time to review your eating habits. Give these habits an "upgrade." This means reducing sugars and processed foods and eating more fruits and vegetables. Consider choosing more organic produce.

2. Find time to exercise, ideally to address stamina (cardiovascular), strength, and flexibility (such as yoga).

3. Review your sleeping habits to improve the quality of your sleep. I'll have more to say about this in pillar four.

4. Practice a relaxation or meditation exercise of ten minutes or more at least once each day. This too will be discussed under pillar four.

RESPONSIBILITY AND SETTING BOUNDARIES

There is one more aspect to developing and maintaining a healthy relationship with yourself: being responsible and setting appropriate boundaries. There needs to be a counterbalancing force to acceptance. If you think of a parent dealing with his or her children (or yourself, dealing with one of your children), you can't be only accepting. You know they can't use crayons on the walls of their bedroom! They can't eat only candy. And they need to get out of bed in the morning, go to school, be present, and do their best. In other words, they must learn to be responsible. At home as well as out in the world, they need to stay within certain boundaries and accept certain responsibilities.

The establishment of boundaries creates a sense of safety for the child. This allows for experimentation and a sense of freedom from danger. The parent must set a balance, with boundaries wide enough to give the child the ability to test and explore while making sure the child feels safe. Too much freedom can be scary or dangerous.

The parent must also establish a sense of responsibility so the child recognizes that to perform well in life, effort and learning must take place.

It is important to establish these same parameters in your relationship with yourself—and for similar reasons. A child whose parents don't establish those parameters might grow up without learning those lessons. One client of mine grew up in an environment that was very constraining. His mother and father were overprotective, holding him back, partly due to their own fears about the world. When he became an adult and left home, he rebelled against their overly protective behavior. He reacted to their constraints by petulantly declaring in his new behavior that no one was going to constrain him anymore. He sought help after two DUIs forced him into treatment. In therapy, he was able to achieve an appropriate balance between a sense of freedom and recognizing the legitimacy of societal and personal boundaries.

In addition to setting boundaries with yourself, it is also important to be able to set boundaries with others—with friends, family, and even in business. So many times I work with people who experience excessive stress in their lives because they have difficulty saying no for fear of being rejected or experiencing someone else's anger or disappointment.

Let's go to step fifteen on The Path to learn these lessons of setting boundaries.

STEP 15 *Setting boundaries*

Let's take two examples of setting boundaries, first with yourself and then with someone else.

With yourself:

Identify a situation in which you are either procrastinating or allowing yourself to engage in behavior that doesn't serve you. This might be something as simple as not going to sleep at a time that would be good for you or putting off important actions that are uncomfortable to do. It might also be not setting healthy boundaries around alcohol or drug intake.

Address this issue by engaging in a dialogue between the part of you that wants to continue this harmful behavior or avoid the actions that need to be taken. The other voice would be the more mature voice that knows what is truly better for you. Take a few minutes to have a dialogue.

With someone else:

Next, identify a situation in which you had difficulty being assertive or saying no to someone. Imagine having a conversation with this person where you take a stand and set a more appropriate boundary. Have a dialogue, with you playing both parts. In other words, respond to what you say as if you were the other person.

When we do this we are sometimes surprised that:

- it feels good to set a boundary
- their projected response is not as negative as you expected
- no matter what that response is, it strengthens your ability to be assertive in the real world

YOUR BILL OF RIGHTS

I want to help you establish the most effective perspective for life. And one of the pieces to this puzzle is what I refer to as your "Bill of Rights." In the Constitution of the United States, the Bill of Rights was almost an afterthought. But it was determined to be so important that it was labeled "Bill of Rights" because those rights are truly at the heart of the concepts of a free society. Similarly, by declaring the following as your Bill of Rights, I'm making the same statement to you.

Go to step sixteen on The Path to read and remember your Bill of Rights.

STEP 16 *Your personal Bill of Rights*

I have the right to:

- Be happy
- Be here

- Accept myself as I am
- Love myself unconditionally
- Feel my feelings
- Set and maintain appropriate boundaries
- Be true to myself
- Love and be loved
- Be treated with respect
- Say no when something isn't right for me
- Be human
- Make mistakes and have flaws
- Do for myself
- Have my opinion and make my own decisions
- Believe in my dreams
- Be vulnerable
- Not always have to be the strongest one
- Experience neuroplasticity

SIGNPOST

- You have been increasing your "Gottman ratio" of positive-to-negative responses to yourself.
- You have let go of a mistake that's been bothering and pre-occupying you.
- You have been "stalking your pattern."
- You have been noting how a healthy internal voice speaks.
- You have taken time to own and appreciate your successes.
- You are more open to accepting the love and appreciation of others.
- You have engaged in an internal dialogue between your old internal voice and the new one you are developing and have addressed self-criticism.
- When you hear your old voice speak, you hear it but listen and react less.
- You are taking time for self-care.
- You are setting better boundaries with yourself and with others.
- You are following your personal Bill of Rights!

CHAPTER 8

PILLAR TWO
Relationship with Others

M any years ago, Paul Simon wrote the classic song "I Am a Rock." "I am a rock; I am an i-i-island. And a rock feels no pain, and an island never cries." Despite Mr. Simon's wishful thinking, few of us live on an island. And we certainly aren't rocks. Yet, according to University of Chicago psychologist John Cacioppo, a large percentage of people are unhappy because of social isolation. And Jacqueline Olds, a psychiatrist who teaches at Harvard Medical School, wrote the book *The Lonely American: Drifting Apart in the Twenty-First Century* because she wanted to bring loneliness "out of the closet." Both of these professionals were struck by the findings from a study conducted by the NORC (National Opinion Research Center) at the University of Chicago, revealing that people reported having fewer intimate friends in 2004 than they had in 1985. And this trend has continued to this day, especially with the internet.

Social isolation just touches the surface of how your relationships with others or lack of them affect resilience. Life is about relationships;

you live in relationship to others, and you engage in relationships on a daily basis. You are, above everything else, a social being! You have work relationships, family relationships, and friend relationships. You have relationships with your car repairman, the person who cuts your hair, and your doctor. And they all have an impact on you.

Most of the time you don't analyze the nature of your relationships. But new research is demonstrating that your interaction with others helps regulate or deregulate your nervous system and your emotions. That's right: Each time you are in contact with another person, opportunity exists for you to experience something positive or something negative. It can be something that enriches you or stresses you—and sometimes stress and enrichment are both wrapped up in the same package. All of these relationships have the potential to trigger emotions—emotions that enrich and foster resilience or emotions that are toxic.

Furthermore, research has also demonstrated that the strength of the bonds of one's relationships is associated with health and well-being. In other words, how close and how safe and secure you feel in your relationships play a role in your health.

The second pillar on The Path is about bringing awareness and health to your relationships, so they support you and contribute to your resilience. And when they are not supportive, you can recognize that and take action so they don't drain your resilience. There is always a tendency to maintain the status quo; but to be resilient, you have to be willing to address relationships that are toxic or otherwise draining your resources without sufficiently giving back.

THE RELATIONSHIP-ENERGY EXCHANGE

There is a quality to the energy that you and others carry and project. If you pay attention, you can feel that quality when you are in the presence of another person. Someone who has a smile on his or her face will tend to "disarm" you. The smile tells you that the immediate environment is safe and you can, to the best of your ability, let down your guard and relax. You might even experience a sense of warmth, which lets you know that a positive flow of energy is taking place.

In fact, research demonstrates that you project electromagnetic signals from your body that are picked up by others in your company. By using sophisticated biofeedback equipment, it's even possible to measure aspects of your heart rate in the brain waves of another person. Someone who is coming from his or her heart, who carries a more coherent heart rate pattern, will positively influence you, your energy, and your resilience. This person will actually make it easier for you to maintain a self-regulated nervous system—a key ingredient to resilience and optimal functioning.

On the other hand, someone who is angry, upset, or simply uncomfortable within his or her own skin will project a heart rate pattern that is more chaotic. We sometimes refer to negative or needy people as "high maintenance," and they tend to be a drain on your energy. Another way of saying this is that they "take more than they give." On an intuitive level as well as an experiential level, we have all encountered people like this who we might say are "stress carriers." In this case, exposure to this kind of energy has the potential to impair your resilience.

Stephen Porges, who developed the polyvagal theory, refers to facial expression and voice tone as our evolutionary defense mechanism that lets us know whether the environment, or a person, is safe or dangerous. We unconsciously pick up a person's energy through this mechanism and it impacts the level of activation of our nervous system.

The second pillar supporting your resilience, very simply, is about maximizing the positive energetic experience, love, and support you get and can expect to get from others, while minimizing the stresses and painful energy caused by other relationships. Interestingly, sometimes we look for support where there is more likely to be pain and stress, and we expect pain and stress where there is the potential for support.

Thus, we might say that the goal is to benefit the most from the good relationships and minimize or even eliminate the harm from the stressful ones. Perhaps most important is the ability to discriminate between these two. In other words, you have to know how to recognize relationships that can be supportive and relationships that are harmful. You want to accentuate the former while limiting the latter. (Red flag: It's important to recognize whether you have a tendency to be attracted to toxic people—critical, negative, moody people—as a result of your primitive Gestalts and what you were accustomed to experiencing as a child. You also want to figure out whether love and negativity were packaged together back then and how that might impact your present. If that is the case, you will have an automatic response you need to be aware of and alter, as it will continually cause stress and tension in your life. More on this later, in our discussion of pillar six, emotional balance and mastery.)

There are two directions to the flow of energy in relationships. There is what you project out to others—and this is your responsibility—and there is what others project and you receive. Here your responsibility is more in your choice of relationships and your ability to block and not absorb toxic or negative energy. In addition, you must not allow others to make you responsible for their feelings.

Let's bring this lesson home by looking at a couple of your current relationships. We will start with those closest to you. This might be a spouse or partner, a parent or child, or one of your closest friends. Let's go to steps one and two of The Path for this exercise.

STEP 1 *Positive relationships*

Think of a person in your life with whom your relationship is mostly positive and without any conflicting feelings. Of course, no relationship is perfect, but think of one that comes close. Take a moment to picture that person in the room with you. Imagine the person in as much detail as possible. Notice how you feel as you picture him or her. Do you find that you're feeling good, feeling calm?

Perhaps thinking about this person puts a smile on your face. You would probably say that being in the presence of this person helps you feel safe and lowers your stress level.

This relationship can allow your body to take a break and restore needed resources, energizing you and enhancing your resilience.

STEP 2 *Conflicted relationships*

Now think of a person with whom you have some conflict. Perhaps it's someone who gets annoyed with you a bit too easily. Maybe it's someone you believe is too critical of you. Maybe it's somebody who leaves you never knowing what to expect. He or she may be nice one moment and upset the next, and you don't know what triggers this reaction. Take a moment to picture this person in the room with you. Notice how you feel. Can you feel a difference? If you check in with your body, you will probably notice some tension and discomfort. This relationship can be considered an energy drain, even if it's someone you love. It's certainly not contributing to your resilience.

You don't often think about maximizing your time with people who have positive energy and minimizing your time with those who are stress activators. Let me say this a different way: There are those whose energy, thinking, and behaviors are positive, accepting, and all about success. Being in their company will automatically lift you and help you focus on positive aspects of your life. When you spend time with negative, complaining, or judgmental people, you will have to work hard simply to keep from taking on that negative energy.

But if you can't or don't want to let go of a relationship that can be draining, there are still resilient ways to continue that relationship.

RECOGNIZE THAT YOU ARE NOT RESPONSIBLE FOR THE FEELINGS OF OTHERS

You are responsible for your own behavior. And when it hurts another person, of course it is your responsibility. But there are many people who want to hold you responsible for their discomfort, their problems, and even their feelings. Frequently, something that you do bugs them. You wind up worrying, "Is he or she upset with me?" "Did I do something wrong?" When you buy into their belief and feel responsible for their feelings, it's called "codependency." Let's be very clear here: You cannot be expected to make someone else feel good! It's not your responsibility, despite all of that person's efforts to the contrary. (You might want to help make another person feel good—but not out of obligation.) When you notice that this is the dynamic of a relationship, it's time to take care of yourself and determine your own set of rules and what is appropriate.

You can't or don't want to get away from some people in your life. But if they are negative, moody, blaming, hypersensitive, or critical, you need some way to block all that toxic energy from activating your body, from causing anxiety, tension, or otherwise making you feel bad. This is not to say that you never do or say something that can hurt another person, and you need to acknowledge that. I will address your responsibility later in the chapter.

The first thing to do with a negative person is remember that you are not responsible for their thoughts or their feelings. You don't have to take on their beliefs or their judgments about you. If they are moody or otherwise depressed or upset, remember that it's generally not your fault. Go to steps three through six of The Path now.

STEP 3 *Protecting yourself from negative people energy*

- If another person is acting strange—say he or she looks angry but isn't saying anything—ask him or her to tell you what he or she is feeling. In other words, take an active step to address your discomfort.
- If he or she is making a judgment or a demand that you believe is unreasonable, let him or her know. In this way, you are being assertive and setting a boundary of what's acceptable to you.

- If you are unable to do this, here is a technique I find quite useful. Imagine a giant glass bell placed over this person. Observe the individual speaking, with the energy created by his or her words having a color and design as the words exit the person's mouth. But as these colored words reach the glass, they bounce back toward the person.
- They can't escape the glass bell. So, as this person talks, the glass bell becomes filled with this toxic energy, but it doesn't reach you. This visualization is particularly helpful in work situations where it may not be appropriate to address the issue.

STEP 4   *Establishing appropriate rules and boundaries*

It might be a new concept for you not to feel responsible for another's feelings, or for you not to feel guilty when certain people give you a look or question your behavior. Identify a relationship in which the other person gets upset with you because you are not doing or responding in a way he or she wants you to respond. To determine what is really appropriate, do the following: Imagine that someone you love and care about—it might be your child or a close friend—comes to you and describes the behavior of this person as if it were happening to him or her. That person asks you, "What should I do?" How would you respond? Working through this exercise usually allows you to be more objective. Thus, you will come up with a more effective way of dealing with the situation.

STEP 5   *Recalling a positive role model*

Let's do another comparison. First I'd like you to think about somebody in your life who is truly supportive and really wants you to succeed. Imagine sharing with them, talking about something that's important to you.

Notice his or her reaction, and then the positive effect this has on you. It might bring a smile to your face. It also helps increase the certainty that what you are doing or thinking about or working on is good.

STEP 6   *Imagining a negative person*

Now let's compare this by imagining somebody who, while perhaps considered a friend, is more likely to be critical of what you're doing. He or she is more likely to find what's wrong with your idea. They are not necessarily doing this to help you sharpen your ideas but because of their insecurities or negative perspective. Again, think about sharing something important and notice how different this experience is.

IMPORTANCE OF REFERENCE GROUPS: THEY CAN PULL YOU UP OR DOWN

What group or groups do you feel you belong to, either formally or informally? Whatever group you consider yourself a part of can be considered a reference group. It might be a particular religious group you are a member of. It might be a gang or a social organization. It might be the Masons or some other organization that engages in different types of activities. Or it may simply be the small group of people you socialize with on a regular basis.

Reference groups can either pull you up or pull you down as they establish conformity patterns. These individuals and groups exert a subtle (or not so subtle) influence on you. They can support and encourage your success and positive behaviors and motivations. Alternatively, the message might be "Don't get too far ahead of us" or "Don't be too nice or different." They can be models for success or models for frustration, excuses, and the status quo.

Most of the time we unconsciously stumble into our relationships and groups. We grew up with these people, met them in high school, or work with them. In any event, you didn't go out and decide *I'm going to look for a critical person or a negative person to be friends with or to hang out with*. It just happened, or you were guided by unconscious patterns that are part of your primitive Gestalt. Go to step seven on The Path now to help you spend more time with people you thought about in step five rather than step six.

STEP 7 *Choosing people you hang with and your reference group*

Take a moment to consider the group or groups you spend time with that can be considered your reference group. Are you satisfied with them, or is it time to look for new associations and people who can be more supportive? If this is the case, here is a process for upgrading your associations, friends, or group that you hang with:

- Make it your intention to surround yourself with positive, thoughtful, intelligent, successful, and caring people.
- Identify current people in your life who fit this description. Make a plan to spend more time with them.
- Make it your intention to take the initiative to go to places, meetings, or events where you are likely to meet the kinds of people you would look up to, people who will be positive models for encouraging your successful behavior.

ATTACHMENT PATTERNS, "MIRROR NEURONS," COMFORT, AND SELF-REGULATION

Recent research is demonstrating that facial expressions of others can trigger specific responses in our brain. There are brain cells that respond based on what is being observed in someone else—thus the term "mirror neurons." These brain cells will fire in response to observations of specific emotions displayed in someone else and have been postulated as the basis of empathy as well as modeling behavior. A loving or caring expression will have one effect, while a frown or critical stare will have another. In fact, according to Stephen Porges, we also unconsciously respond to vocal prosody, or the tone and other qualities of a person's voice. Through a process he refers to as "neuroception" we may become sensitized to certain intonations.

These neurobehavioral processes begin to explain the types of attachments we form while growing up. John Bowlby developed the concept of attachment theory to describe the "lasting psychological connectedness between human beings." This tendency to establish attachment is also believed to be an important evolutionary survival mechanism, as it supports the connections that ensure the care of the dependent child, as well as the importance to the child of this connection. Specific attachment styles are established early in childhood as a result of the interactions and relationship between infant and primary caregivers. This style is part of your primitive Gestalt.

Bowlby suggested that there are four primary characteristics of attachment:

- The desire to be near the people we are attached to
- The drive to return to the attachment figure for comfort and safety in the face of fear or threat
- A sense of a secure base the child can move away from, but always with the knowledge that he or she can return for safety
- Anxiety that occurs in the absence of the attachment figure

In addition, there are four primary styles of attachment: secure, avoidant, ambivalent/resistant, and disorganized or chaotic. These different styles typically derive from the child's experiences in the earliest years of life. Go to step eight now to learn more about your attachment style.

STEP 8 *Assessing your attachment strategy*

Take an inventory of your most important relationships. Imagine each person being with you right now. Do you feel a sense of connection without ambivalence, without hesitation? Or is your affection somewhat restrained?

Do you feel torn between attraction and avoidance? Does thinking about this person cause confusion, as if you are not sure whether to hug or run? How much of this is due to the behavior of the other person? Or do you notice that you have the same style with everyone, even when there is evidence that a secure attachment may be possible?

If this happens, the initial and visceral experience might be stored feelings from the past that are getting triggered in the moment. Sometimes when this happens there is the mistaken tendency to believe they are relevant about the current relationship. Thus, you might keep your distance when it's actually safe to get closer.

A secure attachment is one in which connection to another person is experienced as positive, safe, and nurturing. Being able to establish good, secure attachments will obviously result in greater resilience. This is in contrast to other attachment strategies in which there is either ambivalence or avoidance. These strategies, the result of inadequate child/caregiver relationships, can maintain stress and interfere with the nurturing qualities of a relationship. If you are in a relationship with a person who, at any moment, may be harsh, rejecting, mean, or unsupportive, you waste time and energy putting up your mental guard. Or, if you don't put up a guard, you may get emotionally wounded. Unfortunately, if your original attachment relationship was toxic or impaired in any way, you will be drawn to people like this unconsciously due to the characteristics of attachment, as well as your primitive Gestalt and your drive to complete unfinished business with your childhood relationship experience.

YOUR RESPONSIBILITY FOR GOOD RELATIONSHIPS

I've learned that people will forget what you
said, people will forget what you did, but people
will never forget how you made them feel.
—Maya Angelou, American author, poet, and activist

Relationships are a two-way street, just as there are two directions in which energy can flow. Let's continue with this discussion of good relationships by identifying your own responsibilities. You can't hold anyone else accountable for their words or behavior until you do the same for yourself. By inference, this will also help you recognize when others are acting appropriately for a healthy relationship.

When it comes to relationships, the Golden Rule should always apply: "Do unto others as you would have them do unto you." In the first pillar of resilience—your relationship with yourself—I made two very important points that can be applied here to your relationship with others: (a) it is important to treat yourself with love, acceptance, respect, support, compassion, and care, and (b) the ratio of positive to negative behaviors should be as close to twenty to one as possible. You have primary responsibility to treat yourself in a positive way. I hope you have begun to improve your relationship with yourself, or at least you have begun to recognize when you are not treating yourself positively and know that this needs to be improved.

These considerations hold true in your relationship with others. (If you don't treat yourself positively, you may not treat others that way, and you may not hold others accountable for the way they treat you.) You have a responsibility to do your best when in contact with another person.

There is Dr. Gottman's good relationship ratio of twenty to one: twenty positive comments and behaviors to every one that's negative as the hallmark of a great relationship with others. Of course he was talking about marriage, but we can adapt this concept to all relationships. Again, think about the Golden Rule. You want others to treat you with respect, so it's important to treat others the same way. When the ratio of your or the other person's positive-to-negative behaviors drops below the ratio of five to one, the relationship is in serious trouble. Certainly, it is no longer supporting your resilience or that of the other person. Go to steps nine and ten on The Path now.

STEP 9 *Positive regard for others*

Pick one relationship and think about that person (this can be repeated with each of your relationships). Are you treating him or her with positive regard and a place of acceptance and support? If not, there are two main reasons:

1. You are sitting on some unfinished business with this person. Perhaps some resentment is interfering with warm feelings, or
2. You don't treat yourself in a positive way, and you are simply treating this person the way you treat yourself. You are unfamiliar with a healthier way of relating. If this applies, return to the previous chapter and review how a healthy internal voice or parent talks. Then you can apply that knowledge to this relationship. If you are sitting on unfinished business or unspoken feelings that are getting in your way, it's important to address them if you want the relationship to improve.

I will go into this in more detail when we get to emotional balance and mastery, pillar six. In the meantime, let's do some work on this now.

STEP 10 *Resolving unfinished business*

With a relationship that feels uncomfortable and where you can identify some unfinished business, address this with that person. Follow these simple rules:

•   Find some way of meeting or connecting with the other person. Say something nice about that person or the relationship. This is always a good way to begin, as it establishes a connection and reduces defensiveness.
•   When addressing the conflict, make "I" statements and say how you feel, such as: "When you did such and such, it made me feel so and so." You can't argue about feelings, as there is no right or

wrong way to feel. Make sure you give your feedback in a caring way. If given in an uncaring or insensitive manner, feedback can be perceived as criticism or even experienced as rejection.

- At the same time, give the other person an opportunity to express his or her feelings and be willing to hear those feelings.
- The goal here is for both parties to "hear" or acknowledge the other person and his or her feelings, even if there remains a disagreement.
- Be willing to express a desire to move beyond the conflict.

GUIDELINES FOR YOUR RELATIONSHIP

1. **Always do your best.**
   One of the keys to being on The Path is to always do your best. And in order to do or be your best, you must be present, aware, and in the moment. (FYI: This means not daydreaming and not being preoccupied or worrying about something in the past or future.) Let's adopt this intention in your relationships. It means facing difficult issues with others and being fully present as much of the time as possible. This way of being deepens a relationship. Do your best to keep it positive, supportive, loving, and caring. This will be relative to the type of relationship it is: close relationship, business relationship, or acquaintance.

2. **Don't take things personally.**
   This was one of the agreements in Don Miguel Ruiz's popular book, *The Four Agreements: A Practical Guide to Personal Freedom*. You have no control over what others say or do. Here there are two important considerations: (1) the responses of others come from their own personal view of reality, which is frequently inaccurate and certainly is only their subjective experience, and (2) you cannot get others to think or feel the way you would like them to think or feel. Trying to achieve

the impossible will always create stress and dissatisfaction. The opinions of others are out of your control; the reactions of others are out of your control; you can't satisfy everyone.

3. **Don't make assumptions about the reasons for others' behavior or misinterpret their behavior.**

   You can never know exactly what is going on in another person's head. If you make assumptions, they are frequently what we refer to as "projections" of your own beliefs. You are bound to be wrong. When you don't know and your fantasies are beginning to upset you, the best thing is to get clarity. Ask the other person what he or she meant and what his or her intentions were.

4. **Be clear about expectations and give good and useful feedback.**

   Conflicts arise in relationships when our expectations differ from what the other person is either willing or able to give. Conversely, it can be the gap between what we are able or willing to give and what the other person expects from us. These are the sources of many continual disappointments that interfere with the closeness and enjoyment of a relationship. Take an extra step to make sure that your and the other person's expectations are in agreement.

5. **Be accepting.**

   Think about the Golden Rule. We all want to be accepted. Acceptance is another important key to being on The Path. Therefore, try being more accepting of others.

6. **Be respectful of the boundaries of the other person.**

   If you have a stronger personality than your partner in a relationship, or if there is a power differential, it may be easy to force your will on that person. People in that situation can't say no to you or object to your behavior or suggestions. They might be too scared to stand up to you, or they may simply not be conscious that you are pushing them beyond where they are safe. Ideally, each person should be able to maintain his or her own boundaries, but frequently this doesn't happen. When the other person has difficulty setting boundaries or standing up for himself or herself, it is important not to take advantage of his or her vulnerability. Respect the differences in personal "rhythm" and be sensitive to the other person's state of mind.

7. **Be assertive and set boundaries.**

   One of the hallmarks of resilience is the belief that you can protect yourself. This self-trust reduces your concerns for your own safety. I have seen so many people afraid they would be taken advantage of because they had difficulty maintaining their boundaries or were unable to say no. Some were more concerned about hurting the feelings of the other person than protecting themselves. Remember what they tell you in an airplane: Put on your oxygen mask first, then put one on your child. It is important to know that you will take care of yourself. The result is feeling safe and, thus, experiencing less tension in your body.

   It might even be necessary at times to express your anger in the process of setting a boundary. Sometimes, and with some people, this is the only thing that will stop them. Being assertive will also result in getting your needs met. This, too, adds to your resilience. Finally, if you are able to set boundaries, you will be better protected and, once again, more resilient.

8. **Establish an appropriate level of guard for the person and situation.**

   Setting boundaries and putting up your guard isn't a case of "one size fits all." Too many people are fearful of getting hurt, usually because they have been hurt in the past—be it the recent or distant past—and just want to hide behind a thick wall. This stance in the world actually makes sense if you keep choosing people who are capable of hurting you. But your goal is to be able to adjust the "permeability" of your boundary, so that when it's safe, you are open to receive the emotional nourishment available from others.

You want to be flexible with your guard or defensiveness. If you are with a toxic or manipulative person, you put your guard up so you don't get hurt. But if you are with someone who is more trustworthy (and, of course, this is the goal), you want to be able to adjust and soften your guard. Here is where positive relationships can be energizing and even healing. Being in the presence of loving and caring individuals actually helps your heart function better. Your heart is more likely to beat in a coherent pattern that creates greater heart rate variability, which has been shown to enhance health. The more you can let down your guard with these people and take in their caring energy, the more you will benefit. Go to steps eleven through eighteen on The Path now.

STEP 11 *Self-assessment*

Review your behavior with friends and family and determine if you have been doing your best. Think of one relationship where you have been holding back. What can you do differently? Right now, commit to doing this. Repeat this exercise with your other relationships.

STEP 12 *Shifting your perspective*

Think of a relationship in which there is some conflict. Perhaps you are disappointed in someone. Are you taking someone's behavior toward you too personally?

Do you think that person treats only you like this? Is it possible that he or she treats most people the same way? If you were to let go of your interpretation, how would it change your feelings? Try doing this.

STEP 13   *Where are you making assumptions?*

In which relationships are you making assumptions? Identify one of your relationships in which there is some uncertainty. Look for the opportunity to get clarification by checking out your assumptions.

STEP 14   *Bridging the expectation gap*

Identify a relationship in which there is a gap in someone else's expectations of you. This could be a parent or spouse who expects you to do something his or her way or be more available. The first part of this process is to recognize that the source of conflict is this gap in expectations. Next is to determine what you are willing to give because of your affection for the other person and desire to please that individual while maintaining your own integrity, balance, and boundaries.

Make a conscious effort to address the issue with the other person and be clear about your position. Acknowledge your desire to please—thus establishing the connection—yet also be clear on the boundary you need to set and what you must do to take care of yourself. Finally, recognize that this might not satisfy the other person but that you made an honest attempt to bridge the gap.

STEP 15   *Bridging the expectation gap, part two*

Identify a relationship in which your expectations don't match what the other person is offering—where another person is not meeting your needs. This could be you expecting more from your partner or family member than he or she is willing or able to give. In this case, the best response would be to give feedback to the other person. Enter into an honest discussion while expressing your feelings. If each of you states what you can and are willing to give and what you are not, it will be easier to get resolution. Ultimately, there needs to be a negotiated acceptance so there is a match between what's offered and what's wanted. If you cannot accept the limitations on what the other person can give, this will be a source of ongoing frustration.

STEP 16   *Accepting others*

If you would like others to accept you, begin by making a conscious effort to be accepting of others. Think of one person in particular to demonstrate this behavior to and follow through the next time the two of you are together.

STEP 17   *Being assertive and setting your boundaries*

Think of a person who doesn't respect your boundaries or can be critical, touchy, or reactive. Let's adopt an interesting perspective on this person and your relationship.

Let's say this person has difficulty setting his or her own boundaries and tends to be intrusive with you. Perhaps he or she is a bit heavy-handed or isn't sensitive to the impact of his or her behavior. So you are going to do him or her a favor and set a boundary where he or she is unable to do so. This will make that individual feel better and also improve your relationship. Give people like this feedback; let them know that what they are doing or saying is not OK with you or say no where it's appropriate.

Take a moment right now to imagine a dialogue with this person. Give him or her feedback in as supportive a manner as you can. Then, imagine that person in a chair next to you. Physically switch chairs, and respond as if you were that person.

Take a few minutes to shuttle back and forth between these two chairs and extend the dialogue. How does it feel to be assertive and set your boundaries? Look for an opportunity to do this in real life.

STEP 18   *Making adjustments to your guard*

Review a few of your relationships and consider whether you have made the appropriate adjustment to your guard. Is it high enough to protect yourself from those who can be hurtful? At the same time, is it low enough to receive warmth and love from those who are able to be caring? The next time you are in the presence of others, make a conscious effort to assess your true level of safety, then see if you can adjust your guard accordingly.

DON'T WALK ON EGGSHELLS

Are you ready to address this issue where appropriate? This is one goal of a resilient person.

Walking on eggshells is when the other person gets upset with you too easily, and sometimes you don't even know what you said or did that caused the upset. Usually it's because the other person is hypersensitive or overreactive. I have already touched on many of the issues surrounding this behavior, such as the other person unconsciously expecting you to take care of him or her, or you making assumptions about what he or she is thinking. You may fall into the trap of taking responsibility for that person's feelings.

Walking on eggshells is stressful. It causes tension and worry, and it's distracting. You don't want this in your life! Go to steps nineteen and twenty on The Path now.

STEP 19   *Walking on eggshells*

Identify a relationship in which you feel as though you're walking on eggshells.

Here is one way to handle this situation: Make a decision that this person is simply too difficult, that you cannot try to anticipate all of his or her sensitivities. (There's a caveat here: In your primary relationship with a partner, this is a complex issue. You do have to take some responsibility for not pushing the other person's "buttons"—at least while these sensitivities and emotional issues are being worked on.) You will do your best, but once you decide that you are doing your best, you need to let go, stop worrying, and not buy into the other person's arguments.

Emotional maturity, which comes with full awareness and expression of your feelings, will be addressed within pillar six, emotional balance and mastery. Your personal unfinished business—unresolved issues with mother, father, and other close relationships—will unconsciously interfere with current relationships. For example, unresolved anger—even anger you don't recognize and perhaps deny—will make you sensitive or reactive in the present. You don't want your own unfinished business to bleed into current relationships, just as you don't want this from others.

STEP 20   *Begin addressing unfinished business*

For the moment, consider relationships in which there is conflict or unfinished business. Be aware of this and, where possible, take a small risk and begin discussing the issue with the other person.

COMMUNICATION: OPENNESS, WILLINGNESS TO LISTEN AND TO SELF-DISCLOSE

When we sent a person to the moon, which is about 238,857 miles from Earth, the spacecraft was off course more than 99 percent of the time! How can a mission that requires such precision be off so much of the time? The spacecraft accomplished this feat through continual feedback. The Houston control center was constantly receiving data on its current location from the rocket ship, analyzing this "feedback," then sending midcourse corrections back to the space vehicle. In fact, they refer to this process as an "attitude adjustment."

Just as the spacecraft went off course constantly, disagreements are bound to occur in any relationship. One person's actions will hurt, or in some way bother, the other person. The goal is not to look for a relationship that is perfect or where two people are always in agreement. The goal is to have relationships in which you are able to give feedback that is heard and taken into consideration. When both people are available to listen and make adjustments so that conflicts get resolved and peace and good feelings are restored, a healthy, positive relationship can exist. A relationship of this quality fosters comfort, safety, and, thus, resilience.

So the ability to give and receive feedback is an important requirement of a good relationship. Too many times, the deepening and enrichment of a relationship is short-circuited by a reluctance to address a disagreement. When feelings aren't addressed, there is a buildup of unfinished business, which is accompanied by an unconscious (or conscious) discomfort that gets in the way of closeness. Once created, these feelings need to be resolved. This is how to keep a relationship "clean."

I remember my first group therapy experience. I was clearly green behind the ears and didn't know what to expect. During one of the sessions, a husband and wife got into an argument. Before I knew what was happening, they both had these bats (made of foam and called "batakas") in their hands, and they were whacking each other. They were really getting into it. I was getting tired just watching them, and all I could think was, *Why are these two people still married? They obviously can't stand each other.*

When it was all over, I expressed exactly that. To my great surprise, both husband and wife turned and unloaded their anger on me! They had experienced this as a healthy way for each of them to get their feelings out. Because they had done this before, they knew that their marriage wasn't in jeopardy, and that the process was safe.

I'm not suggesting that every time you are angry at someone you get into the ring with them. But that conflict and those feelings should be dealt with so you can get resolution.

THE TEN (WELL, ELEVEN) COMMANDMENTS OF A GOOD FRIEND

1. Truly want the best for your friend, for him or her always to succeed. Treat him or her that way. In other words, follow the Golden Rule with friendships.
2. Be accepting.
3. Be present with friends.
4. Take equal responsibility for maintaining the relationship.
5. Hold the friend in your heart.
6. Be supportive.
7. Be generous.
8. Be trustworthy by upholding your commitments and expecting the same from others.
9. Don't hold a grudge or hold on to unfinished business.
10. Be clear with your boundaries and expect the same from others.
11. Tell the truth, don't gossip, and don't play games or be manipulative.

THE PATH IS A BLUEPRINT FOR SUCCESSFUL, HEALTHY, AND REWARDING RELATIONSHIPS WITHOUT GUILT OR WORRY

I encourage you to recognize and establish healthy relationships that give you love, acceptance, support, validation, caring, and objective feedback. Begin making the distinction between people who treat you with respect, love, and acceptance; those who treat you inappropriately or judgmentally; and those who create additional stress and tension in your life. Notice that when you follow The Path of healthy relationships there is less stress, tension, and worry in your life. Begin to experience greater joy and less isolation in your relationships by following the steps of The Path.

SIGNPOST

- You are beginning to distinguish positive-energy people from negative-energy people.
- You are beginning to assess your personal relationships: increasing time with positive people and setting better boundaries with negative people.
- You are checking the "Gottman ratio" with people in your life.
- You are noticing the quality of the attachment you have with close friends and relatives.
- You are taking responsibility for improving your relationships.
- You are following the guidelines for good relationships.
- You are addressing unfinished business with your relationships.
- You are following the eleven commandments of a good friend.

CHAPTER 9

PILLAR THREE
Relationship with Something Greater

Our modern industrial society—the world we live in—fosters isolation, as I noted in the previous chapter. Although the Golden Rule is revered, most of the time we live by "survival of the fittest," where it's all about getting ahead or simply surviving, even at someone else's expense. This fosters a feeling of defensiveness. When you are in this mode, the expectation is that others are against you. It may even create the desire for others not to do well, since this makes you look or feel better about yourself. This framework is based on scarcity rather than abundance. And it is the opposite of interconnectedness and a sense that "we are all in this together." It also impairs resilience, because you have a tendency to waste your precious energy on being vigilant.

In recent years this tendency has become magnified by the internet, social media, and the tendency of media, advertisers, and politicians to focus on the negative, what's wrong, and what's dangerous. And because we are primed for survival, we pay attention.

Believing that "it's a cold world out there" and "you can't trust anyone" creates a sense of uncertainty, danger, and emotional distress. The result is a greater tendency to be on guard and to reinforce childhood feelings of personal inadequacy. You'll also have more difficulty letting go in order to recoup from daily hassles and stress.

The United States is very different from other countries, even the other industrial countries of Europe, in the strong belief in individuality; we believe in the "go it alone" mentality and in independence. It's noble to be independent, and it's a sign of weakness to ask for help. This may even be in our genes, as we are the descendants of those who left home to come to America, which demonstrated a certain independence that is a part of our culture. People in our society move more frequently and change jobs more frequently than in other countries or even in our own past. In recent years, and with tightening budgets, there has been less and less of a push to help or consider others. The social safety net has been shrinking. Thus, even for those who are able to take care of themselves, there is still the sense of it being every man and woman for himself or herself.

As I have emphasized throughout this book, The Path is entered more easily when there is a sense of safety and security. The less vigilant and suspicious you need to be, the more opportunity you have to let down your guard and relax. The result is a more balanced use of your psychic energy and an increased ability to turn inward and restore resources used during the times when you must deal with stresses in your life.

This pillar of resilience takes a look at the larger contexts of your life, the world around you, and your beliefs about your place in this world. It addresses the need for and importance of connection that goes beyond your immediate family and friends. Connection and the feeling that there is something more to life, something greater—that we are all part of the same fabric of life—create a sense of reassurance and comfort that helps smooth out the daily hassles, assuage our feeling of being alone, and provide a sense of support and foundation.

I will address three ways in which you can experience a "relation-ship with something greater": first, through spirituality; second, by the identification and development of purpose; and third, by thinking of community and giving service. All of these help reduce the impact of daily hassles and disappointments. The more you can see beyond today, beyond yourself, to a bigger picture and a bigger horizon, the less you are disturbed when something in the moment doesn't go your way. It tends to smooth out the bumps in the road of your life—or, as I would say, it puts you on The Path.

SPIRITUALITY

Einstein once famously said, "God doesn't play dice with the universe." By this he was suggesting that there is an order to life, that things don't happen randomly but with some purpose. The implication is that the purpose or guiding principles are constructive in some way.

At the deepest level, anxiety is the uncertainty of your place in the universe and whether that place is a permanent or temporary location. This "existential crisis," as it is sometimes referred to, lies below the surface of our busy life. It most often goes unnoticed, but it can bubble up when your life calms down. Ironically, when you are stressed by your worries about survival and getting ahead, there isn't any time left over to worry about life or death.

Thus stress, crisis, drama, and business are great preoccupations that put up a smoke screen with the dilemma of your death hovering behind it. Wouldn't it be great if you had this ultimate dilemma addressed? Belief in a loving and infinite existence and universe can do this for you.

Faith and belief may not be positions that can be taught. Further-more, I'm not a preacher whose task it is to get you to believe in God or the interconnectedness of everything in the universe. What I can tell you is that there are significant benefits to holding some spiritual belief, whether it involves God, life hereafter, reincarnation, or simply the interconnectedness of everything. Having such a belief, which is at the heart of most spiritual philosophies, offers a fundamental release from life's uncertainty. This facilitates calmness and, thus, resilience.

SCIENTIFIC EVIDENCE AND SCIENTISTS

Ironically, we are at a time when science is shifting from a Newtonian world to a quantum world. The Newtonian world established the basic principles of physics developed by Sir Isaac Newton and others in the seventeenth and eighteenth centuries. They established the basic principles of the universe. It was the visible universe, taking into account all that was observable, plus forces that were only knowable by their effects, such as gravity.

"Quantum" refers to the minimum amount of any physical entity involved in an interaction. In physics, as it's incorporated into the theory of quantum mechanics, it is the fundamental framework for understanding and describing nature at the infinitesimal level. Without boring you with great detail, there are certain aspects of the discoveries surrounding this field that challenge old perceptions of reality and impact our discussion of "relationship with something greater."

The scientific discoveries of the last half century challenge the existing Newtonian paradigm. The only conclusion to be drawn is that everything in the universe is connected and that consciousness is the fountain from which material things flow, rather than the opposite determination: that ours is a material world out of which consciousness and the mind are just an epiphenomenon. By this I mean that consciousness is simply the result of all those neurons sending and receiving messages.

Lothar Schäfer, a professor and expert in quantum chemistry, notes "that the basis of the material world is nonmaterial." He says that our classical or Newtonian physical world was a separated world. Thus morality was separated from any physical foundation. In a system of separate things, the principles of aggression and selfishness actually govern morality; that's the game. If you can go out and capture a country, do it. "In such a world, you can have a bank make lots of money and ruin the rest of humanity; that's the way the game is set up," he says. Again, this survival-of-the-fittest mentality fosters tension, defensiveness, "me against you," and uncertainty.

In a quantum universe, in which evidence is demonstrating the interconnectedness of everything, morality changes. With interconnectedness, if I cheat him, I cheat myself. This is being brought home more and more, for those who are "waking up," in the notion that we can no longer just spew waste into the environment. Everything has a consequence in the world.

As renowned quantum scientist John Hagelin says, quantum mechanics and the unified field theory bring everything together. At our core, we are one. Take a moment to consider what this means.

SPIRITUALITY AND RESILIENCE

How do these facts influence resilience? In my own journey of discovery and dealing with the stresses of life, questions about death and the nature of this world that I live in consistently reared their heads. It has always been important to me to address the uncertainties in my life to reduce my anxiety and create a greater sense of control and confidence. It also makes me more resilient by nurturing a greater sense of calmness as well as confidence in myself and what I can expect of my environment.

The fear of death is a powerful emotional factor, as I noted. Entire civilizations have perished as their leaders pursued all-consuming efforts to cheat death. One myth surrounding the end of civilization on Easter Island had to do with chieftains harnessing all the resources of their society to build giant statues as offerings to the gods, hoping this would take them to the promised land. It didn't work, of course. However, this foolish and vain endeavor drained the resources of the island, causing the extinction of everything living, and leaving only the statues. To what extent might some of your greatest efforts—perhaps the piling up of "things" such as money or property—be unconsciously designed to put a distance between you and the unknown, between you and death?

ARE YOU READY FOR A PARADIGM SHIFT?

I have always been a skeptic. Perhaps that's why I gravitated to being a scientist. The scientist's mantra is "show me the data." I want proof and valid research if I'm going to change my belief system. About five hundred years ago, civilization went through its last paradigm shift: Galileo and Copernicus demonstrated that we were not the center of the universe, and explorers demonstrated that the earth was not flat. Along with the discoveries of Newton about how the known universe worked, we entered the industrial world with a new belief system. This system explained all the data we had at the time.

Science is about looking at the data and coming up with the most parsimonious theory to explain that data. For millennia, the data supported the Euclidean (from the ancient Greek mathematician, Euclid) and Newtonian picture of the world. This was the height of cause and effect—and linear thinking—where everything was very predictable: If you do this, you get that. If you apply so much force on an object of a specific size and weight, it will go exactly this far. It was a mechanical universe.

But over the past seventy years, more and more data have fallen outside the predictions of this paradigm. At the quantum level, you can no longer predict both the mass of an object and its location in space. Instead, you are left with probabilities. Furthermore, it turns out—and this is a big blow to the objectiveness of science—that the observer of an experiment actually influences and determines the results of that experiment. That's right, there is some invisible influence, a connection between the observer and what's being observed!

Remember we started your journey on The Path with intention. I suggest that intention mobilizes this invisible force between you as the observer and your world. The strength of your intention, therefore, determines its impact on your goals, what you want to achieve.

Work in the area of energy also has shown in countless double-blind studies what the old paradigm cannot explain, such as influence at a distance without any direct physical connection and effects occurring before the cause. Let me give you some examples of this: When I was a professor at McGill University in Montreal, a colleague of mine, Bernie Grad, conducted a series of studies in which he had a healer hold a sealed container of sterile water in his hands for thirty minutes. The healer did not hold a second bottle of water, the control water, in his hands. Barley seeds were soaked in either the healer water or the control water. The seeds were then baked just long enough to injure them and planted, with all other conditions being the same. During the test period, no one knew which seeds had been in the healer's water. The healer, Oskar Estebany from Hungary, had no contact with the seeds.

At the conclusion of the experiment, the pots with seeds that had been watered from the bottles treated by the healer not only had more plants growing in them, but the plants were also taller. This was a double-blind experiment. This means that the person pouring water into the plants didn't know which were which, and the person who counted and measured the growth of the barley plants also didn't know which was which. Remember, what at first seems strange later is considered normal, and we say, "of course." In the same way, our beliefs changed about the world being round instead of flat, and the sun being the center of the solar system, not the Earth.

Another example is a study performed by Dean Radin, PhD, and his associates at the Institute of Noetic Sciences. They tested the effects of two thousand people in Japan holding specific intention to affect water samples located in an electromagnetically shielded room in California. Ice crystals formed from this water, as well as a control water sample, were blindly identified and photographed by an analyst. The resulting images were blindly assessed for aesthetic appeal by one hundred independent judges. Results indicated that crystals from the experimental water were given higher scores for aesthetic appeal than those from the control water. This difference was statistically significant at the .001 level. This means there was only a one in one thousand chance this difference could have occurred accidentally.

In another, just as amazing, study, Radin draped worms over a stick. He attached electrodes to the worms' rudimentary nervous systems. When he shook the stick, it caused a reaction in the nervous systems that his equipment detected. He then did a series of trials in which he would either shake or not shake the stick. The shaking was performed mechanically, and the order of shake or not shake was randomly determined. What he discovered was that the equipment detected a reaction in the worms' nervous system on the trials in which the branch was shaken, but this reaction was detected before the stick was shaken! This cannot be explained within our current scientific paradigm.

For all these years, science has explained away mounds and mounds of data that haven't fit the existing paradigm simply because it was easier to do that than to figure out some other theory to explain the new data. In other words, science did everything it could not to deal with the contradictions to its theories that new data were suggesting.

At this point, science has progressed to the place where our old paradigms no longer fit the data. The Eastern concepts of energy flow can no longer be denied. After all, we don't deny gravity just because it's invisible.

The phrase "people with faith can move mountains" also gives promise to the power of faith. What this suggests is that faith and a spiritual belief can help you reach deeper inside yourself to find greater strength. In the chapter on neurogenesis, I discussed David Bohm's concept about the quantum potential. I'm suggesting that as you reach deeper inside, you are also connecting with the subtle force that permeates the entire universe and is the deepest level of reality. This is where my fourth level of neurogenesis takes place. You are connecting with and being guided by what has variously been referred to as "the source," "the One," or "the Life Force."

CONNECTING TO YOUR DEEPEST SOURCE

When peak performers tap in to their deepest source of strength, I believe this is what they are getting close to. This can become one of your most powerful resources. You are connecting with the unbroken wholeness of the universe, which is The Path of many ancient traditions. The belief that you have this infinite connection actually gives you strength. But more important, it gives you a way and reason to reach deeper inside yourself, which is always the true source of strength, resilience, and success.

When I work with elite athletes, one of the keys to success is helping the athlete be motivated from the inside—the "fire inside," as Bob Seger sang. Athletes have to be motivated by their own inner passion, not the fear of failure or the expectations or judgments of others. When a ballplayer of any kind steps onto a court or field, he or she wants to be focused on giving his or her best performance. That always derives from an inner motivation and is hampered by fear, pressure, or judgments from the outside.

Similarly, your success comes from your own inner foundation. This chapter is not meant to instill any particular belief within you. It is simply to identify factors that will enhance your resilience and success in life. You then have a choice as to how you want to use this information. In science, while we base our theories on research and data, we are never so arrogant as to believe we have all the answers. We have learned much too frequently—in fact, all through the history of science—that existing theories are only our best guess and will eventually be replaced as new data are found to either contradict or expand upon our knowledge. I'm simply suggesting here that a spiritual belief or a belief in the unity of everything will help you be more resilient, and that there is evidence to support such a belief. If you simply make a decision to adopt this belief—just because it's a possibility—it will help you breathe a sigh of relief.

The safer you feel, the more your body and mind can devote their energy toward growth and new brain cells instead of defensive activities. Notice that holding this new belief system, that you are not alone, helps you feel safer and probably calmer. As you hold this belief, you are helping the healing of the hippocampus, which has become damaged by stress, and which is the center of new brain development. Interestingly, whether you truly believe this or not, as you imagine it and imagine that it's true—in other words, take the position of its truth—it will enhance the development of your brain and your resilience.

Spiritual beliefs create a soothing emotional blanket that can surround you and reduce your stress, while enhancing your sense of optimism. Go to The Path and do steps one and two now.

STEP 1 *An imaginary experiment*

For a moment suspend your beliefs and be open to the possibility that what you see is not all you get, that beyond the dimensions you can sense there are many other dimensions—to the world and to life. (Remember, science does not even try to imagine what is beyond infinity or before the big bang.) Imagine now that all these different dimensions and the spirits or energy in these different dimensions are there to support you and your growth. Imagine that, and notice whether it brings a sense of comfort and reassurance to you.

Let's continue with this imaginary story a bit longer. Visualize that in your personal journey, when you make a mistake, when you do something that causes a setback or harm of some kind, that it's just another lesson on your infinite path and journey of growth. As you do this, can you experience a sense of relief?

Just as it is helpful to be supportive in your relationship with yourself, and it's helpful to have relationships with others that feel supportive, a relationship with something greater extends this sense of support, reduces uncertainty, and enhances your basic resilience.

STEP 2 *Extending the experiment*

Let's continue with what we might call a thought experiment, where you are "trying on" a belief system just to see what effect it has on you and on how you feel.

So let's try this right now: Imagine that you are not alone and never alone in the world. There is spiritual energy all around you. And this energy is designed to support you and your continual development. (Come on, play the game; what do you have to lose?) Wherever you are in your own process, this energy supports you and, above all, is completely accepting of you. It knows that whatever mistakes you make will be the source of new learning somewhere down the road.

Take a moment in this thought experiment to completely own this belief system. For the next ten minutes, allow yourself to trust this perspective and do it strongly enough so that it has the potential to exert an effect on you. Now, remember what we talked about in the chapter on neurogenesis—how neurogenesis is possible throughout our lifetime. This, by the way, is also a new scientific perspective. We learn that there are certain factors that facilitate this neurogenesis—or birthing of new brain cells. You can engage this process with this experiment.

Related to this is my own belief that I invite you to take as your own. I believe that I'm in partnership with the universe. You have heard charities say, "We have a matching challenge of $50,000. Every dollar you donate will be matched by this anonymous donor." My belief is that whatever energy I put out into the universe is matched by the universe. If I put out positive energy, I will get that energy back. Conversely, if I'm negative, that's what the universe will send back to me. This has been my experience and provides me with great reassurance.

RITUAL OF INTERCONNECTEDNESS

Rituals that you create and perform on a regular basis can enhance resilience. If they help create order in your life and a sense of comfort, they contribute to your foundation and provide a solid platform from which to act. If they can be tied into this new paradigm I'm suggesting, they will be even more powerful. The next step on the path is a ritual that focuses on your connection with the rest of the universe. It was taught to me by Dr. Liana Mattulich. Perform this exercise at sunrise, facing east, and again at sunset, or as close to that time as possible, as you face the setting sun (or where you imagine it is setting). Go to step three now.

STEP 3 | *Sunrise and sunset exercise and the interconnectedness of everything*

Keep track of the time of sunrise and sunset, which changes from day to day. This exercise will take approximately five minutes.

At sunrise and sunset, take a break from your work and your life. For five minutes, let go of all your problems and thoughts. Face the east in the morning and the west for the sunset, standing with your palms turned up and your hands turned toward each other, right in front of your waist. Feel yourself fully occupying your body. As you breathe in, with palms facing up, bring your hands up—your left hand hugging—sliding up—your body, while your right hand is extended in an arc away from your body and back, as you lift both hands to chest height, and back together.

Next, as you begin to breathe out, extend your left hand forward and out (keeping palm up) and then have it follow an arc downward, back to its starting point, while your right hand, with palm up, slides down your body, again to its starting point. This is the basic movement with your breathing in as your hands rise and breathing out as your hands descend back to their starting point.

I will add one more element to this ritual: Imagine that your right hand, as it goes out and up, is collecting energy from the interconnected universe, and as the right hand comes close to your body and comes down your body, it's distributing this collected energy within you. At the same time, when your left hand is sliding up your body, it's collecting energy from you, your personal energy, and then as your left hand moves out away from your body, you are sending your energy out into the universe. Thus there is a fluid movement of your arms and hands as you simultaneously send and receive energy.

In this process, you are connecting with the universe in a deeply personal manner. You are sharing your energy and best qualities and freely giving of your energy. At the same time, you are receiving the energy of abundance from the giving and loving universe.

Let's add one more aspect to this meditation. For the optimal exchange of energy, I'd like you to think about your gifts, the things that are special about you. As your left hand moves up your body, it collects this energy and your gifts and then sends them out to serve the universe. At the same time, your right hand is collecting what you need from the universe and then brings that in to you.

FEAR OF DEATH

I'm not a sadist. My intention isn't just to make you feel "bad," sad, or scared. In my work, clients don't typically come in because they want to feel sad, angry, or hurt.

I create a strong and accepting container so clients can allow the feelings already inside them to be experienced. Only then can they fully process and resolve existing feelings. By doing this, they are letting go of "excess baggage." Feelings kept inside only serve to distract and constrict. When they walk out of my office, clients feel a sense of relief—they feel lighter, less depressed. In fact, at that point, they are less likely to feel sad or angry.

The same thing can be said about any fear of death. The feelings surrounding this subject get pushed down rather than being addressed. You might ask, "Why address these painful feelings, especially when there is nothing you can do about the situation?" Well, there is nothing you can do about a close friend or relative who has died, but you know it's important to go through a mourning process. Whenever you hold feelings inside, they unconsciously motivate your thoughts, emotions, and behaviors. And as I said earlier, they contribute to depression and anxiety.

Just as there is a process for mourning the loss of a friend or relative, that is exactly the process to use in addressing your own death. Whatever feelings are inside, if they can be recognized and expressed, you will be freed emotionally and become stronger and more resilient. After all, you can't mourn your death after you die, so you might as well do it now.

I don't mean this as a joke or to be morbid. By being present with your feelings about this subject, by bravely facing these feelings, you do a number of things. First, experiencing these feelings helps resolve them. It's the same process that keeps you from mourning the loss of a close friend or relative forever. Instead, after a healthy mourning process, you dwell on the fond memories of that person when you think of him or her—even if those memories are tinged with some sense of loss. Second, by experiencing these feelings, you realize that there isn't anything more that can scare you. Third, by having the courage to face these feelings, you are demonstrating a tremendous strength in yourself. This strength then becomes the source of your courage and self-trust. Fourth, when you stop avoiding these feelings and stop pushing them down, you release all the tension your body is holding from your efforts to keep everything inside. And finally, by fully feeling the impact of your own death, you are also recognizing how precious life itself is. You can use this awareness to renew your intention to make every moment you are alive count and be meaningful. To fully embrace life. Go to step four now.

STEP 4   *Facing your fear of death—helping to make you stronger*

Find a time—about fifteen minutes—to be by yourself without interruptions. Imagine that you are toward the end of your life and will die soon. Allow yourself to feel all the feelings that come up: sadness, anger, loss, fear. Let the feelings move through your body, facilitated by establishing a smooth, conscious, and regular breathing pattern. As you do this, come from a place of acceptance. Here, acceptance simply refers to acknowledging reality and accepting "what is." This facilitates the process. (Note: If you are having difficulty, it may be an indication that you are stuck on either anger or denial. Anger is OK. Allow yourself to express this anger—to God, to the universe, or to the void.)

Notice if your acceptance creates any shift in your experience. For example, some notice that they become less fearful with acceptance. Others find that it makes their sadness less overwhelming.

After you experience your feelings around death, shift your perspective to the awareness that if the loss of life is so painful, it's because life is so valuable to you. And finally, allow yourself to be appreciative that you have life and if it's so precious, you are more committed than ever to fully live your life.

PURPOSE

He who has a "why" to live, can bear with almost any "how."
—Johann Wolfgang von Goethe

I could not imagine living my life in a world where there wasn't any purpose. Each time I have connected with my purpose, it has given me a positive feeling. Whenever bad things happen, I'm able to reassure myself by shifting my thoughts to this long-term reason for living. My mistakes fall more easily by the side of The Path. Identifying and developing a purpose to your life can counter the sense of being alone as well as the meaninglessness of life. But perhaps, just as significant, purpose might have an important biological benefit.

The old belief in biology was that your biological development was strictly determined by your genetic makeup. As with the other areas of science I have already discussed, the "new biology" has demonstrated the primacy of your environment and how the expression of your genes is influenced by your experience. This is a new area of study called "epigenetics," involving how and what influences the expression of your genes and how your nurture influences your nature; also, how your environment and your choices determine new nerve growth and your ultimate development.

But it isn't just about what has happened in the past. The way you live right now, in the present, also determines your genetic expression. Let me take this one step further. If your genes respond to their environment, to how you live your life and to what you learn, then gene expression—the process by which a gene's information develops into cells and tissue—is responsive to your life's purpose.

This is such a powerful concept. It takes the notion of neuroplasticity to new levels. In chapter five, I described the four levels of neuroplasticity. I suggested that neuroplasticity, the growth of new nerve cells, sits at the foundation of resilience. It is the basis of new growth and ties into creativity. So what is new about this discussion?

GAINING COMMAND OVER YOUR BIOLOGICAL CLOCK: PURPOSE, THE ULTIMATE IN USE IT OR LOSE IT

Neuroplasticity neatly ties into purpose and its impact on resilience, and here is how: For the most part, your body is programmed to survive long enough to produce offspring, organisms that will continue your genetic line and carry these genes into the future. For the same evolutionary reason, you are programmed to live long enough to help your offspring survive and take care of themselves. Why is this true? Think about the evolutionary process and survival of the fittest. Once your genes make it into the next generation and your offspring grow up and can take care of themselves, there is no longer a purpose (from an evolutionary perspective) for survival. At this point, the energy of a species—as well as the resources—will be better spent on the next

generation. Said another way, you are programmed, as a result of evolution, for the aging process to speed up once you have served your
species' survival function, in other words, your biological purpose.

This can also be described as "use it or lose it." You know that if
you don't use certain muscles, they will atrophy. The energy of your
body will not continue going into these muscles because the message
is: "The muscle isn't necessary; send the energy somewhere else where
it is needed more." Similarly, if you don't use your brain—if you sit in
front of a TV too long—your brain will get lazy and lose some of its
ability to perform. It will actually begin to shut down. So, when the
organismic imperative for survival of the species is satisfied . . . well,
you get the point.

There is, however, a way to fool Mother Nature, so to speak. Actually, it's not fooling Mother Nature; it's taking advantage of a unique
way that we humans differ from all other species: We are able to create purpose beyond survival. If you have a purpose in your life, you
are giving your mind and body the message: "I have something very
important that I must do, so you better stay healthy and strong until
I complete this purpose." If it's a lifelong purpose, then you will be
imploring your brain and body to stay healthy and function optimally
for as long as possible.

Bruce Lipton, the cell biologist who wrote the book *The Biology of
Belief: Unleashing the Power of Consciousness, Matter & Miracles*, describes
how all the cells of an organism work cooperatively for the good of the
entire organism. By having specific purposes, including specialization
and distribution of function, all the cells of the body work together.
When you establish a life purpose, you are sending a message to every
cell in your body: "Listen up; we have a job to do. You need to be fully
functional and stay healthy and alive so that we, together, can successfully achieve the goals of our purpose." I am suggesting that this conscious message of yours affects your biological clock—slows it down, in
a sense, so you can address your purpose.

There is one more reason to identify and follow a purpose in your life: It gives you direction, beyond simply earning a living or taking care of the kids. Purpose is regenerative, which is at the heart of resilience.

If you already have a purpose, here is your opportunity to declare it and have it work for you. If you have not yet determined a purpose in your life, here is your chance to begin exploring what it might be and establishing one. By acknowledging a purpose and committing to it, you are sending a message to every cell in your body. That message is, "Let's all work together to stay resilient and live a long life. There is work to be done."

To have "purpose" in your life means to extend your horizons. If something stressful, bad, or negative happens today, these negative events will appear more important than they really are if you don't have a clear sense of purpose in your life. If you have a larger purpose in life, you can extend your vision and broaden your horizons beyond the here and now to encompass the "big picture." This helps to smooth out the daily hassles. This aspect of my resilience model helps create a conscious support that can be comforting. Go to steps five, six, and seven on The Path.

STEP 5 *Identifying your purpose*

If you have a purpose in your life—either explicitly acknowledged or implicit in your behavior—identify what it is. Right now I'd like you to declare this purpose. It doesn't have to be perfect; it doesn't have to be completely thought out. Even if it's half an idea, right here and right now, say it to yourself and write it down on a card that you carry with you.

As you do, take a moment to completely own it. Review it when you awaken, throughout the day, and when you go to sleep and hold it dear.

If you don't have a purpose, then the first step is your decision that having a purpose is important, for all the reasons described earlier. Can you establish your intention to find or develop a purpose? If you can, write down a statement at this time about this intention.

STEP 6 *Making a plan*

Make a plan to remind yourself every morning of your purpose and how to follow it.

STEP 7 *Taking an action*

In the morning, identify at least one action you will take that day to support your purpose.

GIVING SERVICE

The notion of interconnectedness also validates the belief that "what goes around, comes around." Said another way, the energy that you send out into the world will have consequences. These consequences will propagate into the world and will also come back to you. In my experience, this philosophy is consistently true. Whenever I have been determined to make something happen, I find a way to engage with the world and with people in the world. I follow my intention with actions. Without fail, shortly after I send this energy out into the world, some form of energy—a result—will come back to me, usually from an entirely different direction.

Life is continually changing. It's impossible to try and hold on to the way things are, to keep things in a static state. It never works. Therefore, it's best to embrace the notion of an ever-changing world. Think of your own body. It must interact with the environment moment by moment in order to keep living. You take in air with your breath, necessary to supply every cell in your body with oxygen. You take in food and water to provide fuel for your body's metabolism.

And then you release into the environment stale air full of carbon dioxide and get rid of the waste when you go to the bathroom. There is a constant flow of energy.

I suggest that giving service is a way to give back for all that you have been receiving! It's a way of keeping the flow going. It's a way of expressing gratitude for the abundance surrounding you.

One way of showing gratitude is by giving back, appreciating what you have by taking some of your benefits and spreading the wealth. If you have been given a gift, sharing that gift extends its benefits. Do steps eight and nine on The Path.

STEP 8   *Experiencing abundance and expressing gratitude*

Recognizing the abundance in the world is a way of establishing the belief that you are OK and that there is more than enough to go around. This addresses one source of fear and anxiety that is the opposite of abundance—scarcity. You no longer have to live under the rule of survival of the fittest!

Take a moment to notice this abundance. It might be within your own home or in your community. It can also be the way you feel about yourself—for example, that you are healthy. Next, express gratitude for what you have. If you are struggling right now in your life, still find something. Give thanks.

Be as sincere as you can be. Imagine your expression of thanks projecting out into the universe. You are sending positive energy into motion. It will have reverberations that are powerful and that ultimately come back to you.

STEP 9   *Sharing your gifts*

The fastest way to encourage positive energy to come back to you, to receive more abundance, is by sending out energy in the form of giving service. Identify a way you can give service sometime during the next few weeks.

Make it your intention to engage in this behavior. It might be volunteering at a hospital or a soup kitchen on Thanksgiving or finding some other local organization to donate time to. It could be joining or giving to a cause you believe in. Write it into your schedule.

BUILDING COMMUNITY RESILIENCE

The final part of this section deals with the implications of working on our relationship with something greater. I'm referring to the benefits of a resilient community. I encourage every one of you to consider contributing to your community and to its becoming more resilient. This means that it can harbor all the qualities I've been discussing: that your community comes from a place of compassion, love, acceptance, and support.

We are all challenged in our goal to become more resilient by the dangers, tragedies, and traumas that surround us. As in our personal lives, we can ignore the pain we observe on the TV or internet, but it nevertheless goes in—deeply. It contributes to the danger we experience, the pain we experience, and the draining of our energy caused by the ongoing activation of our nervous system.

If a community feels that their police are a supporting part of their neighborhood, they will feel more safe. If the leaders of our community reach out and offer understanding of everyone's plight, we feel heard and more connected. These responses can reduce the stress that all members of the community experience.

So much energy is wasted due to a defensive stance toward the world. It contributes to all the illness and impaired emotional and mental functioning I've been talking about. This energy can be shifted, resulting in greater resilience for all the members of the community. We have already discussed sharing your gifts. How can this effort impact the resilience of your community? You begin to impact community resilience by holding the intention to smile and say hello to your neighbors and those you pass on the street. Every one of these behaviors sends a ripple of positivity and acceptance that has an impact. It might even result in others taking your lead and doing the same. Can you visualize what this can result in?

THE PATH

You have completed the first three pillars of resilience. You are also at the end of chapter nine of *The 9 Pillars of Resilience: The Proven Path to Master Stress, Slow Aging, and Increase Vitality*. You are getting clearer as to what it takes to be on The Path and when you are off The Path. If you are taking these steps, as summarized in each chapter's "signposts," you are putting yourself on The Path. Congratulations!

SIGNPOST

- You have experimented with a spiritual belief, trying it on to see if it feels good.
- You are engaging in the "sunrise and sunset" exercise.
- You have explored your fear of death.
- You have identified a purpose in your life or have begun a process to find one.
- You are expressing your gratitude for all that you have.
- You are giving service or exploring how you can give service.
- You are considering ways you can contribute to a resilient community.

CHAPTER 10

PILLAR FOUR
Physical Balance and Mastery

D o you stop to notice how your body feels? Most of the time, you only become aware of your body when it begins to annoy you, when it's trying to tell you that it's not OK, or it needs a rest. This happens when headaches become more frequent, when your stomach feels uneasy too much of the time, or when tension or pain get in the way of falling asleep—or simply relaxing. In other words, you only pay attention when stress and emotional upsets build up in your body to the point where you can no longer ignore them.

As they say in politics, "The buck stops here." I'm referring to how the consequences of what goes on in your life find a home in your body. Everything makes its mark—however small it may be. But over time, these stresses add up. When you sweep stuff under the rug long enough, the piles are noticed even under the rug.

Just one example of this is how stress can affect your appearance. Ongoing release of the hormone cortisol, part of the stress response, degrades collagen. Wrinkles are the result of the weakening and lessening of collagen in the skin.

Consider yourself fortunate if the effects on your body are still below the radar. You may have to look a bit closer to notice the discomfort, the tension, or the fatigue. I'd like you to consider that your body is, in fact, your home. It is your sanctuary. It is the final frontier. When you need to retreat from the challenges of the day, from your life, you want to feel at home in your body. You want to have the ability to deeply relax, retreat, and restore. This process is necessary for recovery, healing, and the maintenance of optimal functioning and performance. Remember, you have no place else to go—or hide. When this is difficult or uncomfortable, that's when we turn to supports such as alcohol, marijuana, Xanax, or behavioral addictions.

EXPERIENCING JOY AND EXCITEMENT

I want to emphasize that our goal is optimal functioning. Think of the range of possible functioning: First there is your normal, everyday behavior in which you are dealing with stresses, daily hassles, and worries. Second, when you take a break, or during the evenings or weekends, you experience some relief from these stresses. When I talk about optimal functioning, however, I refer to the ability to experience joy, happiness, and excitement in your life, not just relief.

Somewhere in your effort to get ahead, as well as your need to defend and respond to danger, the notion of joy and excitement has been thrown out the window. In your efforts not to notice painful emotions, you have constricted or shut down your body; unfortunately, this gets in the way of your body's full expression and aliveness. I refer to this as focusing below the line, where the line represents baseline. Frequently, we are concerned about negative consequences and are simply trying to stay at or return to baseline, and we don't even think about the positive territory of joy and happiness that is above baseline. My intention in organismic balance and mastery is not simply relief or the management of stress and tension: It is the full expression of your body's capacity for excitement. Join me in this pursuit to focus above baseline.

SELF-REGULATION—YOUR BODY'S PRIMARY GOAL

Think of how many times in your day you turn on your stress response. Think of all the situations and people that challenge you and can trigger concern, a sense of uncertainty, fear, and worry, and call into play the activation and self-defense mechanism of your body. This discussion isn't about right or wrong but simply about "what is." Think of your own internal voice that alerts you to possible problems, and the uncontrollable feelings that bubble up to give you pause and cause you to scan your environment for danger.

It can start in the morning when you awaken and worry about what can go wrong—at work, at school, in a relationship. In response to these concerns, your body braces and activates. In fact, your body will brace just going outside your home. You'll encounter traffic, time pressures, and emails requiring responses. Every time you don't have an adequate response for a situation, it triggers your stress response. Even when you do have a good response, your body still needs to mobilize to get the job done.

Now think of this: How many situations or people in your day trigger the opposite—the relaxation response? If you are like most people, there are precious few times in your day that your relaxation response gets turned on. What do you think the consequences are to the frequent activation of your stress response while experiencing only very limited triggering of the opposite, the relaxation response?

At the heart of the mind-body connection is the impact this imbalance has on self-regulation. We are all challenged by the imbalance between the frequency of events triggering the stress response and body activation compared with those triggering the opposite, the relaxation response—the lack of balance between your body going into the protective mode versus the growth and healing mode.

This imbalance stretches the resources of your body and creates wear and tear. Most important, though, it impairs your body's ability to self-regulate. Self-regulation is your body's most fundamental function. Sometimes referred to as homeostasis, it simply means the ability to restore balance and used-up resources whenever situations or events throw your body out of balance or out of tune. This imbalance is like a snowball rolling downhill.

Think of an automobile that is out of tune, meaning that it's not firing on all cylinders. It loses power, it uses up more gas, and it produces more exhaust (waste) as it works less efficiently. Its spark plugs build up crud that further impairs performance, creating more wear and tear on an already stressed engine. An approaching hill becomes more difficult to climb. And climbing a hill while the engine's timing is off causes further wear and tear as the engine strains against its limits and uses the last of its capacity. The result is premature aging and deterioration of the automobile.

Impairment of self-regulation has a cumulative effect. In other words, once set in motion, unless you take constructive action, the impairment will get worse. Some of the mechanisms that get affected were discussed earlier, such as the hippocampus's ability to dampen the stress response. But the problem of self-regulation can affect every system in your body.

Whether we are talking about hypertension, headaches, inflammatory disease, or even cancer and other diseases of the immune system, they all have defective self-regulation in common and at their source. This is what I refer to as Autonomic Dysregulations Syndrome. Numerous studies, for example, show a connection between stress and increased tumor production. Another study demonstrated that people with higher levels of stress take twice as long to heal from a wound than those with low levels of stress. One revealing study showed that a group of accountants' cholesterol level was 50 percent higher around the April fifteenth tax deadline than at other times during the year. Stress also gradually affects both inflammation and cell oxidation, two processes at the heart of disease development and the aging process. For those of you willing to sacrifice your health to get ahead in life, remember that this imbalance also takes a toll on performance, with slower reaction time, greater distractibility, and impaired executive functions of the frontal cortex. Go to steps one and two on The Path now.

STEP 1   *Where do you stand?*

Go to your responses to physical balance and mastery from your Resilience Questionnaire. You want your score to be 10 or higher, in the "optimal functioning" range. Take note of your low responses.

STEP 2   *Reviewing your symptom checklist*

Look at your responses to the Symptom Checklist at the end of chapter one: physical, behavioral, and emotional symptoms. Those items where you scored a 4 or 5 should be highlighted as areas needing attention. However, our goal here is optimal resilience, so we also want to look at items where you scored a 3 or a 2.

Take a moment to note these symptoms. Visualize being symptom free. Imagine how this would feel—being a healthier you. How great would that be?

RESISTANCE TO DOING WHAT'S NECESSARY TO CREATE BALANCE, SELF-REGULATION, AND CALMNESS

It might seem strange that you wouldn't just do whatever it takes to help your body recuperate to maintain optimal balance and self-regulation. But four factors can get in your way, and they frequently do:

1. You feel like you don't deserve it.
2. You feel like you don't have the time.
3. It feels too uncomfortable.
4. It just doesn't happen.

Feeling Like You Don't Deserve

This is a topic that has already been covered within the first resilience and success pillar—your relationship with yourself. Too many of you treat yourselves negatively, still blaming yourselves for past mistakes or taking on real or imagined negative opinions of yourselves from parents or guardians dating back to your upbringing. At this point in the book, you have been working on this issue and have gotten better at being on The Path. Notice if you recognize an improved sense of self-worth while treating yourself with love and compassion and avoiding negative self-talk. It's worth emphasizing this lesson, which will further affect your motivation to become resilient and successful. Right now, let's take another step on The Path and this process. Go to step three now.

STEP 3   *The language of letting go*

Think of something you continue to be upset with yourself about that contributes to feeling undeserving, such as a mistake, a missed opportunity, an inappropriate remark to someone, or simply believing you don't do enough.

Choose something you can no longer do anything about; it's already done. Take a moment, once and for all, to express your feelings with acceptance of reality that the past can't be changed. Get them out, and then let go. Say to yourself: "It's over; it's done; it can't be changed. The best way to make sure it doesn't happen again is to learn the lesson of the experience and then let go.

"Any holding on of an upset can only make it more difficult for me to perform at my best. It's time to forgive myself so I can be more present and more effective." Do this to the best of your ability in this moment.

Feeling Like You Don't Have Time

I saw a cartoon the other day. One executive was saying to another executive, "I save time by not unwinding." Frequently you feel under the gun with so much that needs to be done. Restoring balance and self-regulation seems like just one more chore, one more requirement, one more obligation. When you feel stressed, when you feel overwhelmed, you just try to do what needs to be done, what is urgent. As a result, there is no time to take care of yourself. It's time to change this perspective.

Life is a marathon. It's like a long-distance run. You want to still be standing when you cross the finish line. I mean this literally. You want your goal to be a healthy life right up until the end. This is referred to as "healthspan." In order to do this, in order to stay healthy and to stay strong, it is important to find a rhythm to your life. Taking time to relax does not require a lot of time. Taking time to go inside and recuperate is a requirement not only for your physical health but also for your optimal performance. For every thrust out into the world, you want to go inside and both gather and restore energy.

Engaging in a regular relaxation exercise that helps you restore your body's ability for self-regulation and healing can be achieved in ten to fifteen minutes each day. Can you say you don't waste that much time?

Consider it skill building or training. Your investment in this practice makes you more effective so that you require less time to relax. Right now, decide that you do have ten to fifteen minutes each day for your long-term health and peak performance. Follow the next steps, four and five.

STEP 4 *Making the commitment*

Make this statement to yourself right now: "I commit to taking ten to fifteen minutes each day to practice a relaxation exercise and give my body the opportunity to function optimally." Remember how important it is to stick to your commitments. So, right now, you want to put this time into your schedule. (Also, remember, it is better to do three to five minutes of relaxation than not to do it at all!)

STEP 5 *Getting my free audio download*

Scan the code or go to my website, www.DrStephen Sideroff.com. There you can download a free audio relaxation visualization.

This exercise can be used each day for you to practice restoring body balance.

It Feels Too Uncomfortable

The irony about restoring balance to your body is that the more out of balance you are, the more difficult it is to be present with the resulting body discomfort. If you come to rest when your body is out of balance, the discomfort or tension you experience can motivate you to get moving; it can motivate you to do anything that distracts you from the discomfort. For this reason, we frequently engage in stressful behavior simply to avoid noticing that our body feels stressed and uncomfortable. (Wow, say that last sentence again to yourself.)

Think of a continuum with higher and higher levels of tension as you go up this continuum and greater calm and relaxation as you go down. To begin the process of relaxing, of becoming calm, you must first be present with what is.

This means tolerating and being OK with the level of tension you are experiencing in the moment. When you run away from this, you simply move yourself up the continuum of tension, thereby moving further away from your desired goal of calm and relaxation.

I will give you this guarantee: If you take the time to practice a relaxation exercise—without judgment—you will definitely move down this continuum, entering the territory where your body begins to restore itself. You may not notice this at first. It may take a while to overcome years of tensing in order to begin experiencing the calming effects of a relaxation process; but if you are persistent and have patience, you will be successful. I guarantee it! Please notice the two key words here: persistence and patience. To achieve success, there must be consistency with the process and a lack of judgment. Go to step six on The Path now.

STEP 6 *Body scanning*

Right now, take a moment to stop what you are doing, sit back, and tune in to your breathing. Some of you may be able to quickly go into a smooth breathing pattern. Others may find your breathing choppy, shallow, and/or rapid. In addition, you may notice tension or other bodily discomfort as you become quiet and tune in. This step is simply about accepting whatever you experience in your body. Bring your awareness to the top of your head and notice any tension. Move down through your body, noticing sensations without judgment. Stay in each place for a few moments before moving on. In this manner, work your way down to your feet.

Please keep in mind that I'm not suggesting you stay in this place of calm and relaxation—although you might want to luxuriate in it, once you can achieve it—but simply that you need to take time to relax. In other words, you want to spend time at all levels of body and mind activation and, most important, you want the flexibility to control your levels and be able to relax when you need to and when you go to sleep.

It Just Doesn't Happen

The most common reason we don't take the time to relax and restore is that we simply forget. Even when it is your intention to practice a relaxation exercise, the needs of the moment—the demands that are calling upon you—take priority and help you forget. We are creatures of habit, and your tendency will be to keep doing what you are already doing.

With all you have to do in a day, with all the demands on your time, you cannot rely on your memory—or the feeling to come over you—to do a relaxation exercise. The only way you will be consistent with this practice is by scheduling it into your day. In general, scheduling is most important if you want to establish good habits and be successful. Whether we are talking about a relaxation exercise or any other task that is necessary for your success, it is more likely to get done if you have planned for it and set a time in your day to accomplish the task. I also find it helpful that when you are scheduling something for yourself, you make it just as important as your appointments with other people. Go to steps seven, eight, and nine now.

STEP 7 · *Scheduling to remember and follow through*

Take a moment to schedule a ten- to fifteen-minute relaxation exercise into your day. If you're reading this at the end of your day, put it into your schedule for tomorrow. If you're reading this at the start of your day, you can schedule it today. And each time you do the relaxation, take another moment to schedule your next practice.

STEP 8 · *Getting your personal relaxation exercise*

Again, scan the code or go to my website, www.Dr StephenSideroff.com, and get the free download. Make this exercise readily available for your use.

STEP 9 · *Determining how you will ensure success*

To ensure that you stay on The Path, right now determine how you will make sure you schedule relaxation training time every day.

CREATING ZONES OF SAFETY

In order to let go and to go inside—in order to let down your guard to relax and go into the state of recuperation—you must feel safe. Wariness and hypervigilance can be habits that keep you on guard. Having a sense of unfinished business can also do this. To give yourself the opportunity to deeply relax, you need to create what I refer to as a mental "zone of safety" where you can let down your guard. If your first priority is survival—if you feel any danger—you will not let down your guard and fully relax. It doesn't matter whether the danger is real or if it's just "what if he or she is mad at me?"

You must recognize three levels of safety in order to maintain the most effective energy levels. It's easy to get stuck at a high level of vigilance and activation—you activate for a reason, then stay at that level until the next demand from the environment. Or you are continually scanning your environment, looking for a problem or a danger. In this manner, you gradually step up your energy and tension level throughout the day. Even though you work, take care of your house and your children, and are busy, it's important to be able to modulate and find a rhythm to your energy, alertness, and vigilance during the day.

For most of you, high levels of vigilance are not needed constantly. Your level should be a function of degree of safety, need, and circumstance. Think of your day today, or tomorrow, if you are reading this at the end of the day. Think of the times in which you need to be vigilant. This might have to do with a deadline, a presentation, a meeting, or watching your children. Next, visualize the times during your day when you don't have to be as vigilant. This might be during lunch, or right after, or between appointments. Go to steps ten and eleven on The Path to address the first two zones of safety. By doing this you are also establishing a healthy rhythm to your life.

STEP 10   *First zone of safety*

During the day, out in the world

These are times when high levels of vigilance are not required.

Imagine consciously lowering your vigilance at times during the day when there isn't a danger or a necessity to be on high alert or completely focused. Picture yourself realizing, "I can relax a bit and be calm," even if it's just for five minutes and even if you are still engaged in planning for another event. Visualize letting go of your shoulders, taking a deep breath, and letting the air out slowly.

In addition, visualize actually taking a ten- or fifteen-minute break as well as a lunchtime break and devoting some of this time to letting down your guard and going into a place of calmness. In fact, it's better for your digestion if you create a zone of safety surrounding your lunch and other meals. Just let go and relax. This is a time when you are "off" and not responsible for anything.

STEP 11   *Second zone of safety*

The end of your workday

When you leave work, you want to say, "I'm leaving work, the day is over, it's now evening, and I can relax and take it easy. There is nothing I need to do, and there is nothing I can do until tomorrow morning."

If business is swirling through your head, take a few minutes to sit with a pen and pad or your appointment book. Write down each thought or piece of unfinished business and identify the next step for completion. Write down a specific time in the next few days that you plan to get this done.

If you don't know the next step, write down a time to research what that next step might be. Once you have done all this scheduling, say to yourself, "There's nothing more I need to do this evening. I can let go and relax and not think of any of these things until tomorrow. Now it's time to relax and enjoy my evening and being present with my family."

If you must do some work in the evening, set boundaries, such as 7 to 8 PM, and then hold yourself to this commitment. (Even if you insist on doing work in the evening, there still needs to be a time in the evening when you go through the aforementioned process.)

Establishing a sense of safety is a prerequisite for being able to fully let down your guard and thus achieve deeper levels of calm. It is important to discriminate between an unsafe past and a safe present, and between a dangerous or stressful outside work world and a safe inside world.

Your third zone of safety is established when you go to bed at night. This is the time you need to totally let your guard down. For this to be possible, it is most important to acknowledge that you are completely safe. The greater the sense of safety, the deeper the state of rest you will be able to achieve and the deeper and more restorative your sleep will be. You will also be less likely to awaken during the night. If you have a childhood history of danger or trauma, there might be an automatic tendency to keep your guard up and to feel unsafe. It is helpful to take note of the factors that make you safe right now, such as the security of your doors and windows or that you are not alone. Or that you are a capable adult. It might be necessary to remind yourself that today's circumstances are very different from those of your childhood. It might be necessary, if you have experienced trauma as an adult, again to discriminate between today and the time of your trauma; in other words, to note that present circumstances are different from when you experienced the trauma.

Go to step twelve now to strengthen your third zone of safety. The sense of being safe is also most important when you are practicing a relaxation exercise. You want to set the stage properly. This means, among other things, that you need to clear your psychological space, feel a sense of safety, and accept that there is nothing else you need to pay attention to while practicing the exercise.

STEP 12 *Third zone of safety*

When you go to sleep

Tonight and every night when you go to sleep, make the following statement to yourself: "I am safe. My home is secure. There is nothing I need to do—or can do—to change my circumstance until the morning. In fact, the more I let go, the deeper my sleep and recovery will be. This will result in my best performance tomorrow."

GO INSIDE . . . GO DEEP . . . FIND YOUR HOME

For every effort made out in the world, there must be a foundation. The stronger and deeper your foundation, the further you can "thrust out" into the world. "Stronger and deeper" refers to your ability to internally open, to let down your defenses protecting whatever is inside, including all your feelings and memories. Foundation requires an internal place of safety, and this isn't possible if you are hiding something or trying not to feel your feelings.

You must feel comfortable in your "home" on different levels. Most important, you need to feel at home in your body. It is the ultimate place of refuge. The more comfortable you feel going inside and finding a place of calm, the less you will need to distract yourself from an internal discomfort by staying tense and stressed.

THE ART OF LETTING GO

Take a walk down a busy street. Notice the expression on people's faces and then their posture. Notice the lines of tension, the stooped shoulders. Notice the worry and preoccupation on the faces of so many who walk past you. For over thirty years, stress has been identified by a large percentage of people as the number one problem in their lives. We are continually bracing ourselves for what the world hands us.

For whatever efforts you engage in to be successful in the world—for all your "thrusting out"—there needs to be an equivalent effort of going inside and allowing your body to recuperate, of letting go and releasing the tension. By doing this you are strengthening your foundation.

There is no better practice in the process of maintaining optimal health and self-regulation than giving your body the opportunity to relax. In fact, there are two sides to the equation of resilience: On one side are all the factors activating the body that need to be addressed. This means how frequently, intensely, and for how long your stressors trigger body activation. On the other side of the equation are the forces you bring to bear to turn down this activation. While there are many causes for activation, there is only one single, simple process for turning down that activation: relaxation and letting go. And just as with any other ability, there is no substitute for training and practicing the ability to relax.

Letting go is the opposite of holding on. It's a release. There are many things you can release and let go of. For example, you can release worrying. When you do this, you release tension. You also can release emotions. When you do this, you release your body's need to brace or hold the feelings in. And, of course, you can release tension in your muscles. We have gotten so used to danger that we don't even take note when the danger is not there. I'd like you to consider all the times you are not in danger. Go to steps thirteen and fourteen to continue with the letting-go process.

STEP 13   *The gift of letting go*

Right now, can you say to yourself, "I'm not in danger"? If you are concerned about something that might happen in the future, whether it's tomorrow or next month, can you still say, "Right now I am not in danger"? And if you can say this, then give yourself the gift of letting go. Take a breath and, as you exhale with a big sigh, relax all the muscles of your body. Do this five times. With each exhale, feel your shoulders letting go and dropping and allow your arms to hang from your shoulders like a rag doll. With each breath, see if you can enjoy the experience of exhaling with a sigh and letting go. The more you can enjoy this, the more frequently and the more likely you are to do it.

STEP 14   *Remembering to let go*

To counter the winding up and tensing of your body, establish some way to remind yourself, on an hourly basis, to check in with your body, take a few breaths, and release your tension. If you do five breaths, it will literally take you fifty seconds. What will you use to remind yourself?

YOUR EVOLUTIONARY MISMATCH

Your difficulty mastering stress and self-regulation is compounded by your "evolutionary mismatch." Wow! So in addition to everything else, you need to contend with some evolutionary problem? What will you be hit with next? But wait, instead of worrying about this added issue, let's frame it as "good news" that something that has been negatively impacting you is now being recognized—and then see it as a challenge to use this information to your advantage.

Whenever I have talked about the stress response, I've referred to it as your "fight-or-flight" response, meaning that your body addresses the danger by preparing you to either fight it or run from it. If we go back to our hunter-and-gatherer ancestors of about 20,000 years ago, these were the two ways to escape or defend against any danger. Those ancestors who were most effective had their genetic material transferred to subsequent generations. In other words, we have survived and adapted to be best at mobilizing our bodies for this fight-or-flight response.

But as we have already discussed, few, if any, of your stresses can be handled by either fighting or running away from them. If you are paying bills, working against a deadline, late for an appointment, or in conflict with a family member, you might notice tension in your shoulders or a speeding heart rate. But will this body response help you? This is the mismatch: an outmoded response that is not in tune with requirements for today's stresses and uncertainty, an environmental mismatch. Thus, your body mobilizes, but then there is no release of this energy buildup as you refrain from punching your boss or friend. Instead, by holding in that response, it adds to your tension and overuse of personal energy. Furthermore, if a threatening situation is not resolved, all your body knows is to intensify this same inappropriate response.

What would be a more appropriate response to the stresses, uncertainties, and pressures of your life? If you are in the midst of a time pressure, a problem needing to be solved, or the resolution of a conflict, which parts of your stress response do you truly need—and which parts are depleting the resources of your body and causing damage? Based on this discussion, the first thing you want to do is acknowledge that your life isn't in danger. In fact, the more you can frame the stress as a challenge rather than a threat, the less your body is negatively impacted. This positive and more effective framing of your situation also helps to minimize your emotional reaction, and thus you will be better at maintaining objective and optimal thinking and problem-solving. This is the part of your stress response that truly serves you: being able to focus and concentrate and be present. Next, it usually is not helpful to have any of your muscles tense—whether jaw, arms, or hands. In fact, any task that involves fine motor coordination, such as in most sports—and arts and crafts—you will do better without this excess tension. And finally, it wouldn't be necessary for your heart to pump as hard and as fast as it typically does during stress. These aspects of your stress response will not help you achieve your goals.

REDESIGNING YOUR FIGHT-OR-FLIGHT RESPONSE

To be on The Path, I will help you literally redesign your body's most primitive survival mechanism. This is a revolutionary concept—or rather, an evolutionary concept! That's right, it's time to bring your stress response into the twenty-first century and consciously adapt it to your more civilized demands. Remember that one of the most important characteristics of your brain and body is their plasticity—the ability to adjust, to adapt, and change to new circumstances and requirements. Now we are going to challenge your brain and body to learn a new and more effective stress response that I refer to as a "calm focus." It's not surprising that this is also the objective of elite athletes, because it results in performing at your best.

In order to accomplish this goal, I've designed two different exercises that I'm referring to as my "one-finger pulse exercises." The "one-finger pulse exercise #1" is for deep relaxation, to be employed when you make the determination that you are safe and that it is OK to totally let go. This technique is designed to be used when you are in a zone of safety and can let down your guard. This facilitates the deep relaxation process that you have already been introduced to.

The other exercise, which I'm calling the "one-finger pulse exercise #2," will facilitate the development of a calm focus. This is the new evolutionarily appropriate stress response we are developing. This process should be used when you are engaged in a stressful activity, when there is some danger or threat—or even uncertainty—what I prefer to call a challenge that you need to deal with. In these situations, you want a stress response in which you are focused, alert, aware, yet as calm as possible. This is the new, twenty-first-century stress response! The name comes, not surprisingly, from the use of one finger during the exercise. Go to steps fifteen and sixteen on The Path now to learn these two processes.

STEP 15 *One-finger pulse exercise for relaxation, growth, and resilience*

This is a device to facilitate the deep relaxation training process, to restore body resources, and facilitate optimal healing, growth, and resilience. Turn your left hand palm up. Place your right index finger on your left wrist so that you can detect your pulse (this can be found just below your left thumb, on your wrist). Notice your pulse as you focus on a smooth and deep breathing pattern. Breathe in to the count of four and breathe out to the count of six, allowing your body to relax and let go as you exhale. You might begin to notice that your pulse quickens as you breathe in and slows as you breathe out. This reflects how breathing in triggers the activating part of your nervous system and breathing out turns down nervous system activation. Therefore, you want to spend a bit more time in the exhale mode. This is very healthy and facilitates body healing. Right now, you are connecting with your internal environment. Feel your connection with your hands, your pulse, and your heart.

Let's do a few breaths following your pulse. By breathing in to the count of four and out to the count of six, you are approximating a breathing rate of six breaths per minute. This uniquely challenges your cardiovascular system, encouraging it into an optimal or coherent state. After a few minutes you may begin to notice that your pulse speeds up as you are breathing in and slows down as you are breathing out. That is the indication of coherence and bringing the two branches of your nervous system into balance. Use this technique whenever you are doing the exercise for the purpose of relaxing as deeply as possible.

STEP 16 *Two-finger pulse exercise for calm focus—the new twenty-first-century stress response*

Think of a stressful event you have today or tomorrow. Visualize it, and notice how it activates your body. I would like you to begin learning the calm focus response to address this situation. Imagine being in this stressful experience right now as vividly as possible. Follow the process from the last step but to distinguish these two exercises, let's switch hands and place the pointer and middle fingers of your left hand on the pulse of your right wrist. This will indicate that you are in a stressful situation and that you want to go into a calm, focused state. Notice your pulse as you breathe in to the count of four and out to the count of six. In this exercise, say to yourself, "I want to be focused and alert to handle the stress, but at the same time, I can stay calm. I can achieve just as much, if not more, than if I'm tense." Then go into your optimal breathing pattern while imagining engaging in the stressful challenge. This is a process you can engage in on a regular basis to retrain your stress reaction and help yourself remain calmer under stress.

SLEEP

Sleep is one of the most important body functions that offers us the opportunity to stay in balance with enhanced resilience. During sleep, your body shuts down many of its daytime activities, allowing for the restoration of resources used up during the day. Your body goes through four levels of sleep. At levels three and four, the deepest levels of sleep, the greatest restoration takes place. Neurotransmitters, those chemicals in the brain that facilitate the communication between neurons, get restored during these deep levels of sleep. When this function is impaired, we see increased levels of depression and anxiety, along with many other impairments. New research is now indicating a correlation between poor sleep patterns and developing cognitive impairments. This may be associated with the recently identified glymphatic system, a neuromechanism that helps brain detoxification, but is only activated during deep sleep.

To be resilient, it is important to listen to your body and to be in tune with its needs. For example, fatigue might be the result of poor sleep habits or simply lack of restorative sleep. Steps seventeen through nineteen are designed to maximize the benefits of your sleep.

STEP 17   *Sleeping on The Path and your bedtime ritual*

Imagine that when you go to sleep, you are creating your personal sanctuary, an environment both internally and externally that exemplifies safety, comfort, and peace. It is helpful to create a bedtime ritual for yourself, a process that lets your body know: "We are heading into our personal psychological cave." This includes such behaviors as washing, bathing, skin care, brushing your hair, and other activities that signal your brain, helping to prepare you for bed and going deep inside. It allows your brain to begin turning down the activation level. Identify behaviors you can engage in as your bedtime ritual and plan on doing this ritual every night.

STEP 18   *Adding a visualization*

Accompany your bedtime ritual by creating your own visualization of a personal cave, a psychologically safe environment. Design it to your specifications: a beautiful and comfortable space, with furniture and other elements that give you a sense of safety and pleasure. Perhaps you want to include tapestries that project a sense of warmth. As you lie in bed, close your eyes and use this imagery to add to your sense of total safety and protection, facilitating letting go into a deeper sleep.

STEP 19   *Dealing with your unfinished business*

If your mind is caught up with "stuff" going on in your life—such as business, conflicts, problems—and they keep you from letting go, take this additional step: Make a list of your unfinished business, including what needs to be done and when you will do these things tomorrow. If there is something that is stumping you or that is outside your control, simply put down a time to address it the following day. Then tell yourself: "While I don't know what to do about this, I have a time tomorrow that I will address this issue. Right now, there is nothing more important for me to do than get a good night's sleep so I will be better able to deal with it tomorrow."

Next, shift your focus to your breathing and the "feel" of your body on your sheet and pillow. Allow yourself to enjoy this feeling, as your head sinks into the pillow and your body sinks into the bed. (Focusing on sensations and the "feel" of your head on the pillow shifts your brain from its left-side thinking process to its right hemisphere—helpful for sleep to occur.) By going through this process, you give your brain permission to let go of troubling issues for the night, knowing that you remain responsive to what needs to be done. If thinking while trying to sleep has become a habit, you will find that you keep returning to your thoughts even after doing this. Every time you notice yourself thinking again, consider it another opportunity to retrain your brain, and then repeat the above message and behaviors.

Important: Every time you give in to your thinking and allow it to continue, you reinforce this habit pattern. Every time you stop yourself and refocus on sensations, you are setting new boundaries, making sleep more likely (although perhaps not immediate) and getting on The Path.

THE CONTINUUM OF CALMNESS

For those who have difficulty falling asleep, the difficulty in and of itself can create an atmosphere of fear and anxiety. Wondering "Will I be able to get to sleep?" or worrying that "I'm afraid I won't be able to sleep and I'm going to be exhausted tomorrow" makes it more difficult to fall asleep, as it creates additional tension and activation. Thinking also keeps the left side of your brain activated, when sleep requires the engagement of the right brain. For those having trouble getting to sleep, the path from awake to sleep seems like a giant chasm. We can transform this chasm into "The Path" by thinking of a continuum that goes from levels of activation to gradually increasing levels of calmness and relaxation. Go to steps twenty through twenty-three now to reframe the process of getting to sleep, making it more achievable.

STEP 20 ***The continuum of calmness***

Visualize this continuum as a vertical scale. In fact, right now, notice your level of activation or tension. Check in with your body to do this. Next, place yourself somewhere along this tension/relaxation scale. To help you get to sleep at night, once you place yourself along this continuum or scale, simply set your goal to move down this continuum. To achieve success, all you need to do is move in the right direction, down this continuum.

If you get into bed to sleep and you notice a lot of tension or discomfort in your body, this could be discouraging. "How am I going to get from here to there?"

Again, restate your goal not to get all the way to deep relaxation but simply to begin moving down the continuum. In addition, have patience. It might take a while to start to feel a change. If you begin to judge and say, "This isn't working" or "When will this start working?" this in itself will be activating and make the process more difficult. Instead, say, "As long as I keep doing this relaxation process, I will keep moving down the continuum of greater calmness and eventually notice a difference."

STEP 21 ***Practicing relaxing during the day***

And one more thing: If, after all this, you are still having difficulty and bedtime is too emotionally activating, it may mean that you need to spend more time during the day practicing and retraining your body to relax away from the bed. You may have to become good at it before applying the practice to bedtime. In other words, if anxiety triggered by your bed or bedtime makes it difficult to move down this continuum, start your practices away from your bed and earlier in the day.

STEP 22 *Engaging the right side of your brain*

Let me repeat the two simple ways of helping yourself get to sleep:

Focus on your breathing and focus on the feeling of your body sinking into your bed or your head sinking into your pillow. Both of these approaches shift your brain into right hemisphere activation. Notice the good feelings associated with the comfort of your head on your pillow and having your bed totally support your body as you sink into it.

STEP 23 *Patience and acceptance*

Finally, allow this process to take as long as it takes. Make no judgments. At the very least, you can enjoy the process of letting go and relaxing while you are on the way to sleep.

CONCLUSION

Physical balance and mastery are not about locking yourself up in a monastery to stay calm by avoiding life's stresses. What balance and mastery are about is surfing the daily waves of stress you encounter as a normal part of life, instead of being battered, washed ashore, or drowned by them. It is about finding and listening to your body's rhythms, which tell you when it's a good idea to relax and when you have the energy to keep going. Find your rhythm. Then you can engage in the healthy process of restoring energy used up in the effort to achieve your life goals. The result is attaining better performance and, ultimately, achieving both success and optimal health.

SIGNPOST

- You are taking moments during your day to check in with your body and notice any tension or tightness.
- You are practicing a relaxation exercise on a daily basis, even if you can only do a few minutes.
- You are engaging in this process without judgment and with patience.
- You are identifying your three zones of safety.
- You are remembering to let go throughout the day.
- You are making sure to get a good night's sleep—or working on training better sleeping habits.
- You are becoming more aware of where you are on the continuum of calmness.

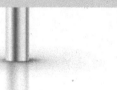

CHAPTER 11

PILLAR FIVE
Thinking and Mental Balance and Mastery

Half this game is ninety percent mental.
**—Yogi Berra, ten-time World Series winner with
the New York Yankees**

know a guy who usually expects—thinks—that something bad will
happen. This anticipation causes him to feel tense, stressed, and worried. When I point this out, he says to me, "I'm only being realistic,"
to explain why he holds the beliefs and expectations he does. He is not
aware that his thinking and expectations are the result of his childhood
primitive Gestalt pattern, and that the results he gets in life are, to a
great extent, caused by these faulty beliefs, which are self-reinforcing.
They filter out what doesn't agree and focus on what validates the belief.

While not everyone would say that he or she is a pessimist, most of
us have a negative and defensive slant on ourselves and the world: what
you expect to happen, how you expect others to treat you, and what

you are able to accomplish. This cognitive or mental strategy—which is usually unconscious—creates unnecessary wear and tear on your body, impairs quality of life and, most significantly, doesn't make you any safer in the world. Research has recently shown, in addition, that pessimism is associated with reduced telomere length. These are parts of human cells that shorten with aging. And despite what you think, your performance suffers as well.

Your brain has enormous untapped potential. How you think can literally restructure your brain (as discussed in chapter four) and improve its functioning for greater success and resilience. However, sticking with old patterns will limit growth and perpetuate current results. This chapter will help you gain control over your thinking and establish the most effective mental strategies, which in turn will trigger optimal brain states that precede mental patterns of motivation and success. At the same time, they will help you let go of fear and anxiety.

NATURE OR NURTURE?

There are two primary reasons for a negative bias. It's not nature or nurture, but nature *and* nurture. From a nature perspective, a defensive bias, or an expectation that something can go wrong or be dangerous, was a good strategy for our hunter/gatherer ancestors, where life-threatening danger was ever present. A more or less constant vigilance was necessary in order to stay alive long enough to reproduce and nurture their offspring. Thus, the genes of those ancestors with this perspective are more likely to have survived from those days to reside in our bodies today.

There are two problems with this: (1) In our civilized world, life-threatening dangers don't lurk around every corner, and (2) today the goal is to live into our eighties and beyond, not just through child-rearing years. How you husband the energy of your body will determine when it will break down. This is what I refer to as the "length of your health." Constant vigilance in life stretches the resources of your body and speeds up the aging process. We could say it shortens your health. These are not just my rules; they are scientific facts, logical and universal truths. Another way of saying this is that being "on guard," always looking for a problem or a danger, takes you off The Path.

As for nurture, if you grow up in a dangerous environment, that is the basic view of the world laid down in your brain. It might be an environment where you could get yelled at, at any time, for any reason; where you were judged; where your parents didn't give you a feeling of safety; or where they were simply experiencing anxiety or stress. This is the blueprint—your primitive Gestalt—from which you view the world. When this is going on, it's easy to have a negative perspective. Even in the most ideal childhood, this bias is fostered as the result of being smaller, less capable, and more dependent than the bigger people all around you.

Those messages from your childhood and the primitive Gestalt blueprint have a gravitational pull. And just like the earth's gravitational pull, they are invisible. But they determined the lines of your growth—and of your awareness and expectations. This is compounded by the fact that the person reading this right now (yes, you) and trying to grasp the conclusion—that you are controlled by your unconscious and primitive rules and Gestalts—is embedded in this very primitive Gestalt! So, instead of being able to direct where your mind goes, you have "a mind of its own." While you might agree and say, "That makes sense," it's going to take a lot more than that to shift this pattern, to shift your center of gravity from your primitive Gestalt to a new mature Gestalt based on true wisdom, with its voice of wisdom.

THE A → B → C MODEL OF HOW LIFE WORKS

It's common to say that someone stressed you out or to feel stressed because you have something important coming up. It's as if there is a direct link: This situation or this person caused my stress. And we tend to blame others or external situations for our sense of overwhelm or excessive stress. In fact, this is not how it works. If *A* is the event and

C is the stress or the overwhelm, then what is *B* in the equation above? If we were able to record and play back the experience in slow motion, we would notice that the *B* is your internal talk, your assessment of the danger—your thinking! If you think that the situation is threatening, you will have a stress response. If you don't interpret the situation as dangerous, you will remain calm.

Have you ever noticed a frown or unhappy look on the face of someone you were with and begun to wonder if that person was upset with you? This might have triggered worry and tension. An assumption—in fact, a fantasy—triggered an unpleasant response in you. Once again the point is that your thinking is an important component of how resilient you are. The more times your interpretations trigger a stress response when it's not necessary, the more you drain your body of needed energy that can lead to body breakdown. Many of your interpretations unnecessarily trigger your stress response. Furthermore, even when there is some danger, it rarely reaches the level of survival; yet it triggers a survival response in your body.

Why is this paradigm so important? Well, if event *A* directly triggered *C*, your survival response, you would be at the mercy of the outside world. Any dysfunctional person who enters into your space (or at least those who mean something to you) would be able to control how your body responds. (And this may currently be true for you.) The good news is that you can take back this control by owning the *B* in the equation. By taking responsibility for your thinking, your interpretations, you now determine whether you will be stressed or not. Taking back control, taking responsibility for your reactions, puts you back on The Path; you will not be as stressed by family members, bosses, or others.

COGNITIVE STRATEGIES THAT GET IN YOUR WAY

While it's great to be able to take back control, if you hold on to the old, primitive Gestalt thinking patterns, you will remain stuck—reacting more frequently than you need to. Over the years, this has been my most difficult task as a therapist: helping people develop a new and more flexible blueprint that is healthier, more adaptive, and the result of new lessons learned, even as they let go of old habits and thinking patterns. The challenge is how to help you be aware of your unconscious guiding principles and way of thinking, be willing to consider new and healthier ones, and then let go of the old, outmoded patterns while adopting the new approach.

Those old rules and lessons were imprinted deep and early, so they feel like they are part of your DNA, part of your basic makeup. The important thing to consider here is that these rules were learned and installed on top of who you are. However, the success that you have achieved—in fact, your basic survival to this point in your life—has become associated with these old defensive patterns and lessons. In psychology, we call this "conditioning." In other words, you have associated your success at getting to this point in life with those patterns. Thus, there is the unconscious fear that if you let go of them, you may not continue to be successful at this level. Worse is the fear that some catastrophe might befall you if you let go of this old, defensive approach to life.

This might seem strange for someone who is struggling to succeed, struggling with a relationship, feeling overwhelmed, or just treading water. But the unconscious fear is that without the old defensive mechanisms, you might do worse; you might drown.

Your old pattern got established because, in fact, it did help you survive as a child. It helped you ignore painful feelings. Where there was abuse, neglect, heavy-handedness, criticism, or lack of love and warmth, then disassociating or numbing yourself minimized the hurt and despair—some of the time. Where there was no hope, because the love and caring you needed from a parent was not going to be there, you created hope by blaming yourself, making yourself the problem, the cause of the lack of real parenting. Creating hope by making yourself responsible allowed you to unconsciously believe, "If I got it right, if I did it perfectly, then maybe I'd get my needs met." Let's acknowledge that it also contributed to patterns of hard work leading to your successes. But this also caused you to blame and dislike yourself on a deep level—to think of yourself as flawed and not OK. It helped get you through childhood (and thus, on one level, you need to appreciate this childhood adaptation). But now, it only gets in the way of your happiness and success.

So, as the first step onto The Path for this chapter, I'm going to ask you to again reflect back on your childhood. In creating and strengthening your foundation, it's important to own your efforts to make it through the struggles of your formative years. It's time to take back your childhood and use the lessons of those years to serve as a foundation for your healthy development in the present. Furthermore, this is a process we need to repeat a few times to overcome all your previous conditioning. Go to step one on The Path now.

STEP 1 *Appreciating yourself for successfully navigating the difficulties of your childhood*

It is important to realize that the faulty thinking and primitive Gestalts that you carry with you today were developed as a learned response to your childhood environment.

Thus, if you can honor yourself for your excellent effort in this adaptation process, it will serve you on The Path.

Right now give yourself some compliments and acknowledgment for your fast maneuvering, learning, and adaptation that got you through the obstacle course of your childhood. Take a moment to pat yourself on the back; yes, go ahead and do it right now. If you made it through a dangerous or even traumatic childhood, this too needs to be acknowledged as a great accomplishment.

Let me identify some of the distorted thinking and faulty beliefs that today can get in your way. One of the most common is to focus on your mistakes and what wasn't done correctly, while discounting your successes and abilities. One of my workshop participants, for example, had a difficult time feeling good about himself. As we explored his history, I stumbled upon one of his successes. I say "stumbled" because, without my questioning, he never would have identified that success. While he worked extremely hard on this project, which resulted in success, he didn't give himself much credit for it.

When questioned, he said, "Well, anyone could have done it. All it required was a lot of hard work." And thus, he gave himself no credit for all his personal qualities, such as persistence, knowing which hard work to do, and making important choices that put him in position for success—as well as being willing to engage in the hard work.

Another participant would find herself experiencing some excitement after success, but it wouldn't last. After the success, she would soon identify something that didn't happen the way she wanted or some minor fault in what she did. Once this occurred, she was off to the races—imagining that others were judging her about this or putting herself down for not doing it right. The success was lost, and she experienced another disappointment: The memory of this success was laid down in her brain as a failure. This also reinforced her negative expectation of future events. Do steps two through six on The Path now.

STEP 2 *Let's look at an example of how you magnify your mistakes and shortcomings while minimizing your successes, abilities, and likability.*

This is one of my most common challenges in working with clients, and I've touched on it in previous chapters because it's so important. Right now, identify some way that you are critical of yourself, have difficulty letting go of a mistake, or are worrying about a future performance.

STEP 3 *Describing the shortcoming you believe you have*

Which shortcoming of yours is involved in your thinking?

STEP 4 *Identifying the qualities you are minimizing*

What abilities, qualities, or other attributes (exhibited in a previous success) might you be minimizing?

_____

STEP 5 *A thought experiment*

Consider that a friend has your identical history and comes to you with this identical situation. What would you be saying to him or her? How would you be reflecting on his or her abilities and previous successes?

_____

STEP 6 *Shifting those positive statements to yourself*

Give yourself this same praise right now. There is no good reason not to treat yourself the way you treat others.

_____

This thinking pattern, the tendency to notice your mistakes and not fully appreciate your positive behavior, will impair resilience as well as your success. So you will experience a 90 percent success as a 10 percent failure. Here the operative word is "failure." Even if you are quite successful, if you misinterpret your success by focusing on what wasn't quite right (perhaps because you are a perfectionist and everything will be less than optimal), the memory will be of failure. This is why so many successful people don't realize that they are successful.

This tendency to disparage your accomplishments can come from many directions. You may have heard your parents talk to you this way. You may have decided or were told that this was the way to improve. It may serve to validate a negative self-image or your personal story. But most of the time it is the result of feeling like you don't deserve. The problem is that with this approach, it will always be difficult for you to develop self-confidence and self-value. Be aware: Any negative bias toward yourself will take you off The Path! It is harmful and will stifle your emotional growth.

OWN YOUR SUCCESSES!

Owning your successes and abilities is not boasting or grandstanding. It is a healthy process to do a self-evaluation, identifying your achievements and taking them in—or accepting them. This process of acceptance is very important. First, when you fully take in any achievement, you actually open to this experience. What I am referring to by "open" is letting down your guard or your defenses, which allows the good experience to be felt and integrated deeper inside you. When this happens you might find, to your surprise, some moisture around your eyes or a softening—what I call "melting." This is sometimes misidentified as sadness. Instead, it's an indication that you are receiving the gifts of your success. When this happens, you are transforming a success and your appreciation of this success into emotional nourishment contributing to the growth of your self-esteem, confidence, and trust in yourself. Do step seven on The Path now. In fact, this is how you gain confidence! This is true alchemy, not turning lead into gold but turning a success into increased confidence and trust in yourself.

STEP 7 | *Taking in your gifts*

Identify a success from your past. Remember it in as much detail as possible. As you do this, allow yourself to experience your gifts and your specialness that contributed to the success.

Remember to breathe slowly as you follow through with this. As you breathe in, imagine that you are owning and opening to this achievement.

At the same time, make sure you don't diminish the process with a "but" or any other qualifications.

In this chapter I am addressing the part of your pattern that resides in your thinking and your expectations. This can also be referred to as your mindset. In my workshops, when I ask who has catastrophic expectations—imagining and focusing on the worst possible outcome—many in the room raise their hands. I then ask, "How many find that you were accurate and that catastrophic results occurred?" Rarely does even a single hand go up.

The amazing thing is that your mental perspective actually influences the results you get in life. A negative perspective or holding onto catastrophic expectations will actually lead to a more negative outcome. And this is in addition to creating more tension and stress.

Research has demonstrated that the way you think affects how your brain functions. Simply reflecting on the process of visualization will illustrate this fact. I encourage people to use visualization to picture the outcome that they want. I use this in my peak performance work with athletes, where I have them visualize taking the perfect shot or making the perfect play.

By visualizing, you trigger brain circuits for that performance that get strengthened simply through this imagery process. But since you are creating this in your mind, you can make every part of your actions perfect. You can consider this a rehearsal that makes the outcome much more likely. (In one study of two groups of basketball players, one group was assigned to engage in the visualization process to practice shooting. Another group went through real basketball practice. At the end of the study, those simply visualizing the practice showed a greater improvement compared with players doing the actual practice.)

But what if you are imagining a negative result? What if you say, "This is going to be difficult"? Or, you think, *I'm not going to be able to do this.* That's right: You are creating and strengthening those circuits in your brain. You are rehearsing for struggle or failure!

You will be less likely to engage in new behavior if you believe danger or rejection is more likely than a positive response. In sports, negativity results in muscle constriction, which affects accuracy. When there are five seconds left in a basketball game, and a player takes a foul shot and the ball clanks on the front of the rim, that's because of tense, tight muscles. Negativity thus impairs performance.

And what do you think the source of procrastination is? That's right, those old, negative thoughts: "I might not be able to do it." "It will be too difficult." "I will get judged."

Simply expecting a negative outcome will trigger all the physical consequences of a real stress incident as well as keep you from being able to relax. This has been demonstrated in brain imaging studies. A continual focus on danger or stress has been shown to literally shrink the hippocampus, one of the most important areas of your brain. I have showed you previously that this impacts self-regulation, pain modulation, and even neurogenesis.

Also, if you expect the negative, it will influence your body language: This can manifest in greater difficulty making eye contact, more agitation, or a less erect stance. You might notice that you get some sort of "feeling" about another person but can't put your finger on exactly what it is. Negative body language is what you are picking up on, and this can influence who gets promoted and who doesn't.

Let's also look at what happens when you have an event slated for the future. Perhaps it's a two-hour performance or an encounter of some kind, and you are concerned that it won't go well. Your worry has two consequences. First, it creates tension. Second, it causes your brain's cortex to shut down. The cortex, the most recently evolved part of the brain, is necessary for creative thinking and problem-solving. Thus you become more tired, less able to sleep and rejuvenate, and can't appropriately prepare for the event because your brain isn't functioning at its best. Do steps eight through thirteen on The Path now.

STEP 8 — *Visualizing something negative*

For a moment, visualize something happening in the future that is negative. As you do this, notice how you feel. Also notice that it creates a negative attraction to this situation. In other words, if the experience is pictured as negative, your tendency is to avoid it.

What I'm suggesting is that if you approach a project, task, or action with a negative expectation, you are creating resistance, procrastination, and avoidance. When you engage in the actions, you will not perform optimally.

In particular, as noted in the previous chapter, worry and distress affect your heart rate pattern. They create a pattern of chaos that further impairs your ability to perform. And finally, when you remember the experience, even if you are successful, you will recall the negative expectation and the struggle.

STEP 9 *Visualizing something positive*

Let's do the opposite right now. I'd like you to think of something that's going to happen in the future, but this time imagine a positive experience and a positive outcome. As you do this, notice the difference in how you feel.

This positive approach and positive attitude foster heart rate coherence, as described in the previous chapter.

This facilitates the optimal functioning of your body. This positive approach produces what I call "positive magnetic attraction."

Your positive expectation actually pulls you toward your goals and toward success.

STEP 10 *Identifying one of your negative self-beliefs*

What negative beliefs—a part of your primitive Gestalt guiding principles—are you holding about yourself? It might be an inadequacy, a "defect," a weakness, or some unworthiness.

STEP 11 *How does this impact you?*

How do you limit or disempower yourself with this belief or rule? For example, do you shrink from challenges or avoid potentially positive experiences?

STEP 12 *How do you limit yourself?*

What boundaries do you set for yourself? For example, how often do you say you can't do something, perhaps even before trying? Or perhaps you want to take an action, but you create resistance simply by saying to yourself, "This is going to be difficult." Another type of limiting belief may be saying, "That's not me." Of course, if you say this, then it never will be you.

STEP 13 *Creating a positive belief*

What positive belief can you identify and shift to? It can be "I can try this and learn from my experience." Or, "When I try something new, it offers an opportunity to learn and puts me in a position for growth and success." And finally, remember one of your positive outcomes to validate having a positive expectation.

ARE YOU ON OR OFF THE PATH?

Unnecessary resistance lowers resilience and shortens your health. Negative thoughts and a focus on the negative create resistance and take you out of the flow of life. When you focus on the positive, you are placing yourself on The Path; when you focus on the negative, you are taking yourself off The Path. Taking in your successes puts you on The Path, while diminishing them takes you off The Path. Where are you right now—on or off The Path?

DO I PROTECT OR DO I GROW?

I referred previously to Bruce Lipton and his book, *The Biology of Belief.* He discusses how cells and humans engage in basically two types of behaviors: protective, on the one hand, or growth and regenerative, on the other hand. I have translated this into either coming from the heart, or coming from *protecting* the heart. Protective behaviors are constricting, closing, walling off the organism from danger. In the case of a cell, this might be from toxins. In the case of you and me, it can be a hostile person or a dangerous situation. But it can also be any time you are feeling some uncertainty. Protective behaviors use up a lot of psychic energy.

Growth and regenerative behaviors cause an opening and a flow of energy. They allow nutrients to move into the organism to restore and regenerate energy. But these functions are inhibited when you are in the protective mode. Thus, positive expectations foster greater growth and a healthy functioning of your brain and your body. I would even say that making the decision to hold positive expectations will result in greater health and performance! This process further validates the opening and taking in of your successes.

One thing I have noticed with many of the clients I've worked with is how negative expectation perpetuates itself. Let me give you the example of one client; let's call her Jane. Jane was an engineer involved in very technical work. Despite her successes and frequent excellent reviews, she approached each new assignment with trepidation. Before receiving the assignment, she worried about whether she would be good enough to respond to the challenge. She would worry that her skills were not keeping up with new innovations. To her great surprise, once she sat with the problem for a while, she almost always came up with good solutions. Furthermore, on the few occasions where she had difficulty, she was able to get help and ultimately work through the problem.

Even though Jane regularly experienced success, what her brain retained was her worry and fear that accompanied that success. The ongoing message she gave herself was how difficult her work was and how fearful she was of the next assignment. This was the memory that got laid down in her brain. And when she was successful, instead of appreciating her abilities and her success, much of the time she was mystified by that success. The consequence of this negative thinking pattern was the maintenance of her belief in her inadequacy, despite all of her successes and positive evaluations.

Many of my clients tell me that they hold negative expectations so they will be less disappointed if things don't turn out OK. Let me ask you: When you have experienced a disappointment or a loss, was it any less painful because you expected it? Let's take a look at these two potential paradigms and the possible outcomes.

Negative Perspective Paradigm: Possibility #1, Negative Outcome

In this scenario you worry about what is going to happen during a future event. You think about the negative outcomes, such as rejection, failure, or loss. During the time leading up to the event, you are tense and preoccupied. Or you worry and may be fearful. You have greater difficulty getting to sleep at night. This perspective also limits your creativity and ability to explore various options, as the worry results in a partial shutdown of your prefrontal cortex. When the event comes and your expectations are fulfilled, what do you feel? That's right; you still feel some type of upset and disappointment, even though you might say, "I knew it." Furthermore, feeling vindicated for your negative perspective predisposes you to feel negative the next time a similar situation arises.

Negative Perspective Paradigm: Possibility #2, Positive Outcome

In this scenario all the preliminary experiences are the same. The difference here is that the positive outcome is experienced as relief and perhaps some good feeling. But typically, what you remember are the stress, tension, worry, and preoccupation you experienced leading up to the event. Thus, despite the success, you retain a memory of the difficulty surrounding this experience, and you also maintain your negative perspective. In addition, you don't use the success to take in a full measure of emotional nourishment to help grow your self-esteem.

Positive Perspective Paradigm: Possibility #1, Negative Outcome

With this perspective, you approach the event expecting good things to happen and expecting success. This opens you to the experience. You are calmer; this facilitates your creativity and optimal functioning of your brain, which makes success more likely. You sleep well, and thus your body is better able to handle the stress. When the event occurs, if you don't achieve your goals, you are disappointed but also more likely to find the positive aspects within the loss and learn from the experience. As you move forward after this event, what sticks in your memory is the positive expectation leading up to the event, as much as the results of the event itself. In other words, the overall experience is not remembered so negatively.

Positive Perspective Paradigm: Possibility #2, Positive Outcome

With this approach, you prepare and hold positive expectations as in the previous scenario. With the successful outcome, you fully enjoy and take in the experience. The result validates a positive outlook and expectancy, adding to your sense of self-efficacy and self-esteem as well as a sense that the world is abundant and nurturing.

YOUR CHOICE

After reviewing these scenarios, which makes the most sense to you? What mental strategy do you think would help you most on your path, and which would result in greater resilience? For many of you, your very success has become the training ground for your worst habits. You are fearful or worry about an outcome . . . and then the catastrophic expectations and negative outcome don't happen. While this is not a conscious association, essentially what your brain receives is, "Wow, every time I worry, every time I imagine terrible things happening, it turns out OK!" Whether you are aware of it or not, you are telling yourself, "Worry, because then things turn out OK." In fact, the truth is that you are successful in spite of your worry and anxiety. It's time to break this superstitious connection. It's time to choose a positive expectancy.

Remember, carrying a positive expectation doesn't mean you can't plan for all possible results, including the negative. You simply don't have to dwell on the negative once you have worked through how you would handle it. Do step fourteen now.

STEP 14 | *Fostering a healthy attitude and positive expectation*

This calls for the creation of an affirmation about your mental expectations. Please take a moment to create one in your own words. It can look something like this: "I plan for all possible outcomes, but I expect to achieve success in all my activities."

Or "When I have an event, decision, or performance in the future, I expect it to turn out well; I expect a positive outcome."

Write this down on one of your three-by-five index cards. Add it to the affirmations you read and meditate on when you awaken, reaffirm at least three times during the day, and repeat before you go to sleep.

EXPECTATIONS ABOUT A HOSTILE WORLD OR THE LESS THAN HONORABLE BEHAVIOR OF OTHERS

Negative expectations have different sources. They might stem from doubts about your own abilities, or they might result from a belief about the intentions of others or that the world is more hostile than friendly. Furthermore, if you make poor choices of companions or business partners, you are even more likely to maintain negative outcomes and expectations.

Again, it's important to begin this discussion by realizing that you come to this belief due to childhood lessons and your childhood environment. If your childhood environment was dangerous, you will come to believe that the world is dangerous. If either of your parents was critical and judgmental, you will believe that people out in the world are going to judge you and be critical of you. If your parent said one thing to a person's face but the opposite behind his or her back, it will make it difficult to take in praise or to trust what your parent, or anyone else, says to you.

These beliefs are further strengthened by your choice of relationships. Since you tend to gravitate toward people who are familiar, you will choose those who treat you similarly to your childhood experience. This tendency will validate and strengthen childhood beliefs and leave you more resistant to change.

A broad range of childhood experiences can lead to an interpretation of danger. For example, if you have a parent who is anxious, the message is that there is some danger—after all, why else would she or he be anxious? If a parent is preoccupied with business, bills, or his or her own inadequacy and thus is less available to you, as a child you wouldn't have said, "Oh, I understand why my mother can't give me the nurturing and reassurance I need. She is just too busy or stressed." What happens unconsciously is more like, "There must be something wrong with me that my mother isn't taking care of my needs. I need to be better or do more to be good and to get her attention." Or you might just decide to give up. This impacts your view of yourself as well as your view of a world that doesn't meet your needs. Go to steps fifteen and sixteen now.

STEP 15 *Exploring your expectations*

What childhood experiences can you recall that fit this discussion?

In what ways did you experience your environment as being dangerous, or at least uncertain and not secure? What behaviors of either of your parents gave you the feeling that you weren't OK or that he or she didn't trust you to make the right decisions?

For example, an overly protective parent might convey the message: "I don't trust you to take care of yourself, so I have to watch over you more closely."

STEP 16 *Shifting your internal dialogue*

What would be a more positive message you can now begin giving yourself? Write this affirmation down on your three-by-five card for regular review. Be on The Path right now and take this step.

ARE YOU CONTROLLED AND AFFECTED BY THE JUDGMENTS OR NEGATIVITY OF OTHERS?

A common theme is how people stop themselves from engaging in potentially enjoyable and successful experiences because they are afraid of the judgments of others. For example, consider the person who is dying to get up and dance but doesn't believe he has enough rhythm or doesn't want to look foolish. Or the person who avoids taking actions to advance her career because she fears being judged. This is particularly true of women in business. In addition to concerns about their abilities, they worry about not looking feminine.

One of the hallmarks of resilience is not being controlled or affected by outside negativity. The peak-performing athletes and executives I work with are always focused on their own abilities and not what others are thinking. Remember, the only person you have true control over is yourself. Whenever you hesitate because you fear the reaction of others, you are putting your life and your success in their hands. It's time you put your life in your own hands. This is taking responsibility for your life. This is being on The Path. Go to steps seventeen through twenty now.

STEP 17 *When do you worry about other's judgments?*

Where are you being stopped in your life out of concern about the judgments of other people? What is the judgment you are afraid of? Is it "You look silly," or you look too "this" or not enough "that"? If any of those subjective judgments really were being made, is it worth it to stop your own growth to prevent people from thinking about you?

STEP 18   *Imagining ignoring the judgments of others*

Imagine that you are not held back by your fantasy of others' judgments. Imagine instead that you take action on something you have been avoiding. Imagine how freeing this would be. Visualize the positive outcomes you achieve by taking this action. Right now, engage in a dress rehearsal.

STEP 19   *Being able to say, "I deserve"*

Do you feel you deserve that positive outcome? You need to be able to say yes here. If you are having trouble, go back and do some of the work in chapter seven about your relationship with yourself.

STEP 20   *Taking action*

Now make your visualization from step eighteen into reality! Make a commitment and a plan to do one behavior that, up to this point, you have hesitated to engage in due to concern about judgments.

It's not only your actions that can be affected by the negativity of others. If you are not careful, you may unconsciously absorb this negativity. This creates unnecessary physical stress and tension. Whenever a negative person is in your presence, he or she is projecting his or her physiology into the environment. You are part of that environment. As mentioned previously, it is possible to detect the heart rate of others in your own brain wave patterns. What do you think the chaotic heartbeat pattern of the negative person is doing to your brain waves? Go to steps twenty-one and twenty-two now.

STEP 21   *How are you affected by negativity?*

Think of a person in your life whom you would characterize as being negative. How does his or her negativity affect you? Perhaps you notice a dampening of your mood. Perhaps you become a bit anxious. Perhaps the negativity takes away the excitement you were feeling.

STEP 22   *Overcoming the negativity of others*

Neither you nor the other person benefits from your absorption of negative energy. So this is what you must say to yourself: "I'm not helping this person by getting down like him or her. I'm only perpetuating the negativity.

"Instead, let me demonstrate a more positive demeanor and be a model for this other person. Let me set the tone of the interaction." When you take charge of yourself like this, it will also interfere with and minimize the absorption of the negative energy.

MASTERING YOUR THOUGHTS AND DEVELOPING A POSITIVE MINDSET

Whatever your perspective, it is important to have control over your thinking. This means when you go to sleep, you are able to turn off your thoughts. When you want to be present and in the moment, you are not distracted by worries or thoughts about what you need to do, what you did wrong, or what someone else might be doing. In other words, you want to have mastery over your thoughts as well as your thinking patterns, so you won't be distracted and your thoughts won't be a source of worry or anxiety.

The fast pace of life, the way you are bombarded every moment by new and different stimuli, has a direct impact on your brain. This quickness of change leads to the conditioning and adaptation of your brain—a good example of neuroplasticity—to want this fast pace and to want and expect frequent change. This causes your mind to wander and makes it difficult to stay focused when you need to be. Thus, there are two ways you lose control over your thinking: (1) troubling or fearful thoughts intrude on you, and (2) your brain can be easily distracted, impairing focus and presence.

The good news is that these interfering habits of your brain can actually be unlearned in the process of training to achieve better, healthier patterns. Let's take interfering thoughts first. I will address being easily distracted when you get to pillar seven, presence.

There are many reasons you hold on to and keep returning to troubling thoughts. The most frequent include:

1. You are worried about, or expect, a potentially negative situation or outcome in the future,
2. You are upset by some unfinished business in a relationship, and
3. You are still upset with yourself about a mistake you made in the past.

The next steps on The Path will address each of these issues.

Your "mind-body" always wants to address and finish unfinished business. This was the finding of Gestalt psychologists in the early part of the twentieth century. One of their classic studies separated subjects into two groups. One group was fed a full-course dinner, and then participants were shown an abstract painting. The subjects were asked what they saw in the painting. The other group was deprived of food for five hours and then shown the identical abstract painting. Members of this second group, the deprived group, all recognized something food related in the painting—every one of them. But not a single subject who had just finished eating saw food-related items in the painting! The psychologists concluded that these findings demonstrated how organismic needs organized and motivated people's approach to their environment.

Since it's impossible to have closure on something that hasn't happened yet, we have a tendency to keep trying to resolve or at least reassure ourselves about events in the future. Thus, it is easy to find yourself caught in a loop, envisioning various scenarios and becoming nervous each time you picture a negative outcome. When you address future possibilities, it's important to make a distinction between productive planning and ongoing worry. Yes, you want to plan for all eventualities: What will I do if this happens? But once you plan for potential outcomes, it is time to let go. At this point, any additional thinking can be referred to as worry. Worry drains you of your psychic energy and speeds up the aging process. Your energy is better spent on more productive activities. As Bobby McFerrin sings, "In every life we have some trouble. But when you worry you make it double." (Now sing with me: "Don't worry, be happy.") Do steps twenty-three through twenty-nine now.

STEP 23 *Future worry*

Identify something in the future you are worrying about. It might be next week or next month. If nothing comes to your mind, think of something you are at least concerned about so you can engage in this process.

The first step, if you have not already done so, is to make a plan: Determine what you can do to ensure success and when you will take these actions. Do this right now. Next, think of the negative outcome you are worried about. What would be the best action you can take if this happened? Now you have made a contingency plan for what you are worried about.

STEP 24 *Next, make the following statement to yourself*

Say to yourself: "I have done whatever planning I can do to prepare for this future event. I have or I will take whatever actions are part of this plan. There is nothing more I can do at this time.

"Any additional thinking or worrying will only create unnecessary stress and tension and leave me less capable of optimal performance in the present moment. And the most important thing to ensure future success is being fully present and functioning optimally right now."

STEP 25 *Unfinished business*

Again, any unfinished business is a source of agitation and distraction from the present as you unconsciously try to finish it in your head.

The first step is to identify what is unfinished. In the next pillar of resilience, emotional balance and mastery, I will address unfinished emotional business.

Right now, let's address situations, commitments, and other projects you have procrastinated or otherwise left undone. What is the first action you need to take?

STEP 26 *What is the obstacle?*

What's getting in the way of you taking this action? Is there uncertainty as to the best action to take, or are you afraid you will be unsuccessful?

STEP 27 *Identifying additional information you may need*

If there is uncertainty, will additional information help you make a decision? If so, what is the next step in order to get that additional information? Plan on taking this step.

STEP 28 *Can you accept not taking action?*

If you are afraid of failing, making a mistake, or making the wrong move, consider the consequences of not taking action. Are you satisfied with the result? If you are satisfied with the consequences of not taking action, then decide right now that this is how you are achieving closure—by letting go of this unfinished business. But if this isn't OK with you, then . . .

STEP 29 *Taking action*

It is important for you to take action. Here is resilient thinking on The Path to make it easier to take action: (1) Your positive mindset is that if you take action, you're already successful, because (2) even if you make a mistake, it's an opportunity to learn from the situation so you will have greater success the next time. Furthermore, you are demonstrating courage, a source of self-trust.

THE DEVELOPMENTAL PROCESS

Part of being on The Path is recognizing that change usually occurs incrementally. It's a step-by-step and trial-and-error process. But if you are impatient, expect to get it right immediately, or become uncomfortable when this process is awkward, it will interfere with your growth. In my own childhood, I remember helping my father build things. I was very eager to do what he was doing. "Dad, let me try," I'd say as I watched him hammer a nail into wood. So he would give me the hammer, and I'd start hammering, hitting the nail first in one direction and then in the other. After a few whacks, my father would become impatient, take the hammer from me, and complete the process.

The unspoken and unintentional messages I received from my father were: It's not OK to make a mistake or be awkward, and I didn't do it well enough. In my adult years, I realized that the result of these lessons was that I didn't want to try something unless I knew I'd get it right. And I felt I should do it perfectly, right from the start, even though this was completely unrealistic. Development always involves trial and error, awkwardness, and learning from mistakes. So it needs to be OK that you make mistakes. The story goes that Thomas Edison failed one thousand times before he created a working light bulb!

Language is also very important in your success. For example, in preparation for handling a life challenge (notice I avoided the word "problem"), the simple statement "That's hard" will make achievement of the task more difficult and can result in procrastinating or even giving up prematurely. Our mental habits reinforce our old patterns while interfering with new brain cell growth.

If you want to have a more positive mental approach, it cannot be accomplished immediately. Just like other types of learning, this ability needs to be developed through frequent attempts and ongoing effort. (This awareness alone will help the reader who typically feels hopeless when he or she tries to change and has difficulty doing so.) This series of steps will outline the approach to becoming more positive and being able to let go of nonproductive thinking. This four-step process includes: (1) noticing the nonconstructive thoughts, (2) offering a cognitive rationale for letting go of these thoughts, (3) going through a process of centering, and (4) switching to a more positive mental frame of mind. Go to steps thirty through thirty-three now.

STEP 30 *Awareness of your present mental approach*

What part of your mental approach is negative or otherwise interfering with growth? Reflect on how you look into the future and your typical expectations.

STEP 31 *Rationale to let go of negativity*

Give yourself a strong rationale for letting go of this thinking pattern and adopting a more positive approach, based on the ideas I have presented in this chapter.

STEP 32 *Centering yourself*

Take a moment to center yourself. This means focus on your breathing, feel yourself connected to your chair and the ground. Be fully in the space that you are occupying. In other words, be fully present and interrupt any wandering of your mind. Feel your strength.

STEP 33 *Holding a positive expectation*

What is a more positive mental approach for you to hold? Be specific, such as "I can expect a positive outcome." Transfer this positive mental approach to one of your cards.

IN CONCLUSION AND FOSTERING A GROWTH MINDSET

Your ability to think is one of your most beautiful and unique characteristics in the entire universe. You can use it to create, imagine, solve problems, and learn. Your thinking has many dimensions, each of which enriches your life incredibly. Good thinking patterns will put you on The Path, but each dimension of thought also has a dark side—the potential to send you off track or off The Path. Your thinking leads the way in your life, but it can also set you back. Where you place your focus determines where your mind follows. So many of those I work with keep hurting themselves by minimizing their successes and overemphasizing their mistakes. Commit to being more positive in life. This approach is also in alignment with the notion of a growth mindset as opposed to a fixed mindset. A growth mindset means that you have the power to grow out of any harmful thinking or judgments, that recognizing any shortcoming is an opportunity to learn a more effective approach. With this way of living, you free yourself for unlimited potential.

I want to conclude this chapter by reviewing the four "cognitive balance" questions from my Resilience Questionnaire:

1. **"I am not bothered by the judgments of others."**
   Trying to please others takes the control of your life out of your hands and adds to uncertainty and stress.

2. **"I don't dwell on mistakes."**

Dwelling on a mistake—something that has already happened—magnifies the impact that mistake has on you and your life. It distracts you from being present, hurts your confidence, and makes you feel less capable walking into the future. It is imperative that you follow the process in this chapter to work through and let go of anything you are carrying from the past, particularly your mistakes. Letting them go leaves you more available to fully experience the present moment. This makes it more likely that you will be successful.

Remember, if there is something you really feel bad about, cultivate compassion toward yourself for the mistake. If this is difficult for you to do, imagine that someone you dearly love made the mistake and visualize how you would respond to them.

3. **"When I wake up in the morning, I worry about what might happen during the day."**

Planning your day, anticipating what might go wrong—as well as what might go right—so you can prepare for it is healthy. Any additional thinking can be called "worrying." This is simply a waste of psychic energy that can be put to better use. Worry takes you down the road of burnout without any benefits. You may have inadvertently developed the belief that worry helps you in life, but this is an error in thinking, as discussed earlier in this chapter.

You can address this issue by repeating these arguments to yourself and then switching your focus to the potential positives for the day. But perhaps more important, here is the optimal framework for your day. Begin each day by saying: "This is (fill in the date, say it's January 1, 2025). It's the only January 1, 2025, that I will ever have. It's my responsibility to make the most of this day and to do my best to enjoy it, learn from my experiences today, and feel good at the end of the day that I fully participated in life."

4. **"I am usually on the lookout for what can go wrong."**
    Your two goals are resilience and success, or they can be stated
    as success with good health. Focusing on the potential posi-
    tive experience will help you lean into your life and embrace
    it. It will help you stay calm and keep your brain functioning
    optimally. This is much more beneficial than having negative
    expectations.

SIGNPOST

- You are appreciating how well you adapted to your childhood environment, even if these lessons are interfering with your current life.
- You are taking in the successes in your life without adding a "but."
- You are identifying some of the qualities demonstrated by your successes.
- You are visualizing and practicing positive expectations about upcoming events.
- You are identifying some of your existing negative beliefs and artificial boundaries that have been getting in the way of your success.
- You have begun shifting to more positive beliefs, expectations, and a more healthy attitude.
- You are creating positive affirmations about yourself and your expectations.
- You are overcoming your fear of the judgments of others.
- You are developing a positive and growth mindset.

CHAPTER 12

PILLAR SIX
Emotional Balance and Mastery

Nothing ever goes away until it teaches us what we need to know.
— **Pema Chödrön, author and Buddhist teacher**

ll humanity is passion; without passion, religion, history, novels, and art would be ineffectual," declared novelist and playwright Honoré de Balzac. And Johann Wolfgang von Goethe said, "All the knowledge I possess everyone else can acquire, but my heart is all my own." According to Carl Jung, "There can be no transforming of darkness into light and of apathy into movement without emotion."

Emotions are wonderful. They are what make life worth living. We yearn for our heart to pulse with passion and love, and if it doesn't, it's because we have been emotionally wounded. We want a beautiful sunset to take our breath away. And again, if this isn't the case, it's because our spirit has somehow been stepped on. Emotions give texture to our lives. And emotions can open us to the deepest parts of ourselves.

Yet emotions can also be terrifying. And for many people—either consciously or unconsciously—fear or discomfort surrounding emotions can create barriers to the full experience of life and even cause havoc. Those of you who want to control your emotions—who don't want any surprises or uncertainty, who are afraid of dropping into the depths of depression—will wind up exactly where you don't want to be by avoiding and suppressing your emotions. What you are avoiding will remain, but you will unconsciously create an entire additional level of pain and life disruption.

Emotions are a jealous master. You ignore them at your own expense; they will make you pay. Fritz Perls, cofounder of Gestalt therapy, said that depression is simply "the depressing of emotions." I would add that anxiety is frequently the bubbling up of feelings you are afraid to experience and are trying to run away from. I say "run away" because some of our stressful behavior is motivated by unconscious discomfort with those strange sensations that begin to surface during times of calm.

ANXIETY AND YOUR RELATIONSHIP WITH FEELINGS— "HE PUSHED MY BUTTONS"

Rarely are we taught about our emotions and the best way to deal with them. Instead, we are more likely to have observed inappropriate behavior surrounding emotions—ugly fighting, denying, and feelings getting hurt—much of the time, without any resolution. Emotional discomfort can be triggered by something in your environment or by uncomfortable sensations inside yourself. When the discomfort comes from inside—due to old, unfinished business—you busily scan your present environment to identify a danger that is not there. You believe the internal discomfort is a trusted signal that there is danger. The result is often ongoing tension and anxiety.

As a child, you didn't have the capacity to fully deal with your emotions; they could be overwhelming. You were dependent and didn't have the external or internal resources to handle those emotions. As a result, you learned various ways not to notice your feelings. This was adaptive as a child, when it was important not to get overwhelmed. But now, as an adult, it has negative consequences: You learned to hide feelings, and that lesson continues to interfere with the awareness of and resolution of your feelings in the present.

A previous workshop participant said to me, "Why should I want to feel these unpleasant feelings? They should stay buried; that's where they belong." I explained to him that the anxiety he was dealing with was caused by those unwanted feelings bubbling up to the surface of his awareness. His fear, that they would burst through and he would lose control, was the source of his anxiety.

Emotions are a normal and important part of life. Yet many people are uncomfortable with their emotions and tend to avoid them. They make us feel vulnerable, uncertain, and out of control. Unfortunately— and much to the surprise and chagrin of most—when you ignore or otherwise stuff feelings down, they stay with you and there are consequences. Every time you find yourself overreacting, it's probably an indication you have touched into some emotional unfinished business; your "buttons" got pushed.

EMOTIONAL HOLDING PATTERNS

It's not possible to simply decide—either consciously or unconsciously— not to feel. At the root of the word "emotions" is "motion"! Emotions motivate and activate your body. First discussed by Wilhelm Reich and later developed by Alexander Lowen into body therapy approaches such as bioenergetics, the "holding in" of emotions is necessarily accompanied by tightening or tensing of muscles, which Reich referred to as "body armoring." This process facilitates the holding in of emotions and the process of not noticing them. This body armoring contributes to muscle aches and pains, and it also interferes with the flow of energy through your body, as the tightening reduces flexibility. When this is chronic, it has health consequences as well as interfering with joy and pleasure, as your body can't properly build and then discharge energy. This difficulty can interfere with the flow of sexual energy as well as reaching completion in business. Your body loses its vitality, its resilience. Check it out: Look at yourself in the mirror. You can see the signs of your bracing in the lines and creases in your face.

BEING IN HARMONY WITH YOUR EMOTIONS

It's thus important to be in harmony with your emotions. Emotions need to be your friend, and you should feel OK experiencing them. When this is true, you open yourself up to greater joy and passion in your life.

How do you know that you're in harmony?

- You are able to be calm and stay calm without pushing your emotional energy down.
- You are able to resolve and let go of emotions and emotional events easily and quickly.
- When someone else is upset, while it might concern you, it doesn't make you tense.
- Activated emotions in your body do not keep you awake. You fall asleep easily and sleep deeply.

A healthy relationship with your feelings and dealing with them appropriately is crucial for resilience.

Here are a few signs that you are not in sync with your emotions:

- You have reactions that appear way bigger than the situations that trigger them.
- You sometimes feel like your feelings are in control, not you.
- It's difficult to ever get over some feelings.

- When you have a feeling, you are uncomfortable and want to move away from it.
- Your feeling is as likely to be anxiety or depression as anything else.
- You wonder if your feelings are right or wrong.

I remind clients who want to ignore their feelings that this does not make any difference as to whether they are there or not, and it doesn't make them go away. It just makes clients less capable of dealing with and resolving their feelings. In fact, being aware of and addressing your feelings is the only way to make them go away.

When feelings are not appropriately dealt with, they will unconsciously control your behavior and your life, as part of you is always trying to resolve what's unfinished. This will lead to depression or anxiety and can take the color out of your world. It also impacts your ability to be focused, and it's responsible for type A and other inappropriate behavior in which there is a continual push to do more and more.

It's interesting how emotions, such as sadness, have gotten such a bad rap. It comes from the lessons of our childhood and the efforts of parents to have their children avoid pain. Growing up, my relationship with emotions developed based on my family's consciously avoiding them. I grew up with the unspoken message: "Stay away from 'bad' or uncomfortable feelings." My mother would make up little white lies so that feelings would not have to be faced. Later on, I realized that my parents were very uncomfortable with their own feelings and thus steered me away from mine. My parents interfered with the major emotional experiences of my childhood. Thus, when I visited my grandfather in the hospital as he was dying from pancreatic cancer, I was told he was going to be all right. I was very close to my grandfather, and this lie deprived me of the opportunity to say goodbye and tell him how much I loved him.

Step onto The Path in this chapter on emotional balance and mastery by examining your relationship with emotions. Explore the following questions as your first five steps on The Path in this chapter.

STEP 1 *Who pushes your buttons?*

Who pushes your buttons? Is it a parent? A child? A partner? What about at work?

STEP 2 *How do you react?*

What happens when you get activated? What change do you notice in your body? Do you notice how it throws you off balance? And then do you automatically go into an emotional reaction that may not give you the best result?

STEP 3 *Describing your relationship with emotions*

How would you describe your relationship with emotions? Do they make you feel uncomfortable? Do you avoid them in order to not feel vulnerable or "unnecessarily sad"?

STEP 4 *What are you holding on to?*

Do you have feelings that are difficult to let go of?

STEP 5 *What has been left unfinished with someone close to you?*

Are you aware of holding on to feelings toward someone close to you?

YOUR AMYGDALA AND THE POWER OF FEAR

Freud and his colleagues were early proponents of the profession of psychology, which tries, among other things, to discern what's going on inside the mind. Many years later the behaviorists came along. They described the mind as a black box, something that was impenetrable. If you can't see what's inside the box, they decided, then the focus should be on observable external behaviors and responses. Next came the humanists, who said what is inside is important even if you can't see into the box. Today we have overcome the problem of the black box—to some degree. We now have tools, methods for scanning the brain that detect such things as localized blood flow. We can literally see what's going on inside the brain and which areas are getting activated.

An important discovery is how the small area of the brain referred to as the amygdala lights up when there is danger. This amazing area of the brain is our alerting mechanism. Of all the areas in the brain, this is the one that seems never to forget. This is understandable because it's your survival mechanism. If you encounter a serious danger and survive, you want to be alerted as quickly as possible when you encounter something similar in the future. You also want to react as quickly as possible. Thus, the response from the amygdala will interrupt the slower processing of information that goes up to your cortex, where reason lies. In this nucleus, any past trauma, dangerous situation, or other threat is remembered. It will be triggered, and the amygdala will light up whenever something is indicative of danger.

Survival is your most important consideration. You are biased toward making an error on the side of overreacting, over expecting. When the amygdala activates, it wakes up the entire brain and prepares you to deal with danger. Your entire body goes on the alert. The way we get caught in this ruse is by believing there really is a danger due to old associations that are no longer relevant. And you will be convinced of it.

When your amygdala expects something dangerous, you don't think clearly (remember, activation of the amygdala occurs before messages can get to the cortex for you to do a bit of reasoning). Thus, you tend to be more rigid in your perceptions, your thinking, and your problem-solving. You lose your cool because you have less access to your "executive" brain. Here is what intrepid, stranded fictional sailor Robinson Crusoe had to say about fear:

"Oh, what ridiculous resolutions men take when possessed with fear. It deprives them of the use of those means which reason offers for their relief. The fear of danger is 10,000 times more terrifying than danger itself, when apparent to the eyes; and we find the burden of anxiety greater, by much, than the evil which we are anxious about."

This last statement is so true of our feelings as well: Our fears of noticing or experiencing our feelings will always be much worse than the reality. Nothing can compare to your fantasies. Do steps six through ten now.

STEP 6 *What triggers your fear?*

Which people or situations will trigger your fears, perhaps even before you have time to think about it? Do you find yourself fearful of the judgments of others? Perhaps there is some fear as you meet certain people or a group of people?

STEP 7 *What is your fantasy?*

What is the worst thing that could happen in these situations?

STEP 8 *Reality check*

If you told this to a close friend, what would he or she say? Would your friend be more likely to agree with you—or to say that your fears are ungrounded?

STEP 9 *Does fear create safety?*

Does your fear and worry make the situation any better or any safer?

STEP 10 *Accepting the worst*

If the worst did happen, would you survive?

DEPRESSION

Data from the National Comorbidity Survey (NCS) indicates that approximately 16 percent of the population suffers from major depression. But even this large percentage doesn't take into account those flying under the radar: those just not happy in life, unmotivated, and burnt out. When you take this group into account, the number probably doubles or triples. This prevalence is not because people are born depressed or have the "depression gene," but because of the consequences of suppressing their emotions. Numbing is a way of avoiding feelings, and it's a process you learn very early in life. Unfortunately, you aren't able to selectively numb just the bad feelings. Suppressing your emotions also takes its toll on your ability to feel joy!

It's time to do what's necessary to move on. It's time to finish your unfinished emotional business.

The expression "time heals all wounds" turns out to be untrue. Wounds do not heal, and emotions cannot be released until they are appropriately addressed. When feelings are not addressed or released, there is a buildup of unfinished business. Since we have an unconscious drive to complete unfinished business, a part of ourselves is always split off or distracted in its efforts to reach completion. These distractions affect focus and concentration, and they ultimately cause us to be less present. Finally, as noted above, holding in these feelings affects our musculature.

And because we unconsciously want to protect our wounds, we create protective shells around these areas of emotional pain. They then become "no-man's land" within our delicate psyche. There may be areas within yourself that you can identify: perhaps a hurt caused by criticism from a parent or spouse, or the apparent lack of caring or attention from someone close to you. This results in holding patterns that interfere with breathing and many other physical functions of the body. They can lead to headaches and other physical symptoms. Most important, these holding patterns interfere with the flow of energy throughout the body. This is a major cause of depression and your inability to experience joy.

If you are old enough you might remember the Winston cigarette commercial on TV. It included a jingle, repeated over and over: "Winston tastes good, like a cigarette should." After repeating this jingle perhaps ten times in thirty seconds, the last time it played, it stopped at "Winston tastes good like a . . ." Listeners spent the rest of the day trying to finish that darn phrase, thus keeping the name "Winston" in their heads.

Unfinished emotional business is any emotionally charged experience you haven't had the time, ability, or awareness to work through. What's unfinished might be from yesterday, last month, last year—or from your childhood. As you try instead to unconsciously protect your wounds, you develop "scotomas"—blind spots. Emotional balance and mastery is about getting in touch with these feelings and finding some way of "finishing" them: expressing, getting them out, and then accepting and letting go. The result is the shedding of excess baggage you no longer have to carry around wherever you go. This is associated with a freer flow of energy and a greater ability to be fully in the moment, where life truly occurs. It is The Path to overcoming anxiety, depression, and many of your fears.

VULNERABILITY

Many of my clients think of being vulnerable as the dumbest of ideas. "Why would anyone want to be vulnerable?" said one of them. "It's just too scary. Who knows what can happen?" And, of course, there is the danger of getting emotionally hurt. But this perspective fails to recognize the benefits of allowing yourself to be vulnerable. First, the vulnerable state of being open is necessary in order to fully receive positive energy from your environment. That includes a loving comment from a close friend or relative or acknowledgment in your business or social circle. When your guard is up, it may protect you, but it also interferes with your ability to receive positive energy, compliments, and emotional nourishment.

The second potential benefit of vulnerability is that it's only in this state of openness that you can touch the deepest part of yourself. This touching in to your deepest self with positive feelings is tremendously rejuvenating.

Being vulnerable is scary and uncomfortable for two reasons that result in putting your guard up. Armoring serves to protect you from the slings and arrows of the outside world. It can also block uncomfortable messages from inside—by this I mean your feelings.

Sometimes it's appropriate to protect yourself from the outside world. Your level of guardedness should be variable and determined by the level of danger in the moment. So, at work, it's appropriate to have your guard up, to some degree. But at home and with friends, you want to be able to let your guard down. In other words, you want flexibility to adjust your guardedness based on your environment. But in any event, ultimately it doesn't serve you to block your awareness of your internal environment—your emotions.

YOU DON'T HAVE TO BE A MASOCHIST TO FEEL YOUR EMOTIONS

The notion of getting in touch with your feelings is not masochistic. It is not about causing or creating pain. The idea is not to manufacture emotions but simply to allow those that are already inside to come to the surface. Resolving unfinished emotional business is about identifying feelings and what they are about, finding some way to express them, accepting them, and then finally letting them go. This process will set you free, as the saying goes.

Another way that we get stuck resisting the process is either a sense of loyalty or a sense of ambivalence toward, say, a parent you are angry with. For example, many of the people I work with see a parent who, when they were a child, was abusive or overly critical and judgmental, and that parent is now old and feeble. That parent no longer looks or acts anything like the angry or critical person of the client's childhood. "How can I be angry at him or her—look how fragile he/she is?" Or, "He isn't that way anymore." We might even go into our heads and rationalize, "He/she did the best he or she could." Or perhaps the parent one minute showed love and the next minute he or she was mean. So you say, "Well, but he/she did love me."

It is important at some point to accept and let go, to remember that love or other positives were in play. But much of the time we do this prematurely, before we have fully addressed and released all our feelings. When you go to the dentist to get a cavity fixed, he or she doesn't just cover the decay with a filling. The first thing that's done is the removal of the decay, so there is a good foundation for the new material. The same applies here: You can't fully let go of the past until you deal with all the buried feelings.

Another way that some of us get stuck is by being afraid to confront the person you have feelings about. "I don't want to confront my father; he will get even angrier than I am toward him." "I don't believe my father will listen to me, so what's the use?" Or, "If I ever confront my mother with my feelings, I'm afraid she will never speak to me again."

These are certainly reasonable concerns. In fact, if completion of your unfinished business required acknowledgment or even just being listened to by the other person, you would be stuck. After all, the only person you truly have control and responsibility over is yourself. And many of you do get stuck waiting, hoping, and praying for the other person to listen to you, accept you, appreciate you, and give you the love and attention you deserve. Furthermore, these expectations are impossible if the person you are upset with is dead or is otherwise no longer in your life.

The good news is that you don't need anybody else to finish your unfinished emotional business. Receiving the hoped-for response is not the goal of the process. (While this would be nice, you need to look elsewhere to satisfy these important needs in a healthier way and with people who are capable of meeting these needs—to be discussed later in the chapter.) Instead, it is the feelings you carry inside that need to be finished. Finishing simply means being aware of your feelings, allowing yourself to feel and experience these feelings, expressing these feelings, and finally accepting what is and letting go. Accepting "what is" doesn't necessarily mean you like it—or liked what happened when you were a child. It's simply the recognition that you can't change the past or the other person and must accept reality—this is the way it is.

Many people I work with will tell me that they have done this—perhaps with numerous previous therapists. "I've expressed my feelings till I'm blue in the face, and I still can't let go of this anger." What interferes with letting go is the hidden or unconscious need for the past to have been different or for the other person to be different. "I deserved better." "I can't accept that I had such a horrible childhood." Or, "I'm just trying to understand how they could treat me that way." Any time we want the past to be different, which is impossible, or to understand why it happened, we are grasping at straws and refusing to accept. Some behaviors just can't be understood and don't make sense. This inability to let go is what keeps us stuck and keeps the frustration and anger going, as if in a revolving door. It's the refusal to fully accept the loss—and thus to fully feel the emotional pain—that keeps you in limbo. You become a prisoner of these impossible wishes—a continual drive to get resolution of old emotional issues.

An example of this is a sixty-five-year-old man who was still resentful of his mother and her intrusiveness in his life. The intrusiveness went on during the client's childhood as well as his adulthood. As a result, he carried this sensitivity and anger into new romantic relationships with women. Only after fully feeling and expressing the anger and then sadness about the original relationship was he able to let go and be fully in the moment with the new women he met.

Often, finishing an emotional experience does not require the involvement of any other person. People can finish emotional business with those who are no longer in their lives or who are no longer living. You can also finish this business with those who are still in your life but otherwise unavailable. When you appropriately deal with emotions and let go of them, you no longer overreact or misdirect your feelings. You are more capable of staying on an even keel. The result is a healthy flow of energy in your body and a greater ability to relax and experience joy, along with greater resilience.

You may be among those who have learned to hide your emotions even from yourself. This is a part of your defense system, causing stuff that is uncomfortable to get submerged below your level of awareness. In other words, you have developed some very sophisticated ways of not noticing. For others, these pesky emotions intrude too frequently into your life, causing havoc or annoyance.

On The Path in this chapter, you will learn to be a detective and keen tracker, stalking your prey. In this case, it's your primitive Gestalt pattern, your emotional unfinished business. One of the primary ways you become aware of emotions you have held inside is by experiencing reactions out of proportion to the triggering situation. This is a clear indication you have a pool of feelings inside that has just been tapped. Another way is to notice that you don't feel comfortable being warm to a close friend or relative. You might be wondering why you don't simply feel good when they are experiencing success. In fact, you might be wondering why you don't simply feel good when *you* are experiencing success. This might indicate that you are holding angry feelings or negative judgments of yourself.

The next steps on The Path will help you identify your unfinished business. This will be followed by a dialogue in which you speak to that person in absentia and express your feelings. Be aware, however, that completing unfinished business does not involve trying to change the past, make someone different from whom he or she is, or make someone else apologize or even hear what you have to say.

It is about first acknowledging feelings that need to be expressed and released. Next, it is about recognizing what the feelings are about. This is followed by expressing the feelings in whatever way is most possible for you. Don't get caught up trying to get the other person to hear you, to apologize, or to turn back the clock to make the past better. One of my clients, who grew up with a cold, negative, and abusive mother, had great difficulty acknowledging her feelings at first and then expressing them. She would say, with tears, "She's the only mother I had." Another client felt it would be disloyal to even consider having anger toward his father. The key here is that—as much as you might want to have a good and loving relationship—if you are harboring anger, it will get in your way. Hear that: You will be more able to experience love when you acknowledge and release the anger. The more you address and let go of unfinished business, the more you are moving onto The Path. Do steps eleven through twenty on The Path now.

STEP 11 *Identifying your unfinished business*

Identify some excess emotional baggage or unfinished business you are carrying around. Who is it with? How is it affecting you?

STEP 12 *Visualizing the other person*

(The following steps can be repeated with all your primary relationships—and even others with whom you might be aware of having some conflict. I suggest starting with a person close to you. However, you might want to ease into this process by starting with someone you are less attached to.)

In your mind, select a person in your life, someone with whom you suspect or know that you have unfinished business. Do this when you are alone and won't be disturbed.

Let's bring in the empty chair, as we have done in previous exercises, and imagine this person sitting in the chair, in the room, in front of you. Take a moment to picture that he or she really walked into the room and sat down opposite you.

Visualize that person in as much detail as possible. As you do this, notice what happens in your body.

The process of imagining allows for a true experience of being with this person and causing your feelings to rise to the surface. At the same time, since the person isn't really there, you can express whatever it is you need to without worrying about hurting someone's feelings, making them angry, or causing him or her to reject you.

This process also helps activate the brain circuits associated with these emotions and this person. This makes the appropriate memories more available for modification. Simply look at this person and notice which emotions come up.

STEP 13 *Becoming aware of your feelings*

Continue to notice the feelings that arise and identify them.

STEP 14 *Becoming aware of what the feelings are connected to*

What feels unfinished? It might be anger or frustration for what this person did or didn't do. What would you like to say to this person?

STEP 15 *Accepting, having no expectations*

Remember, the goal is to identify and finish your unfinished business, which is usually emotional. Completing this unfinished business is about expressing it—for the sole purpose of getting the feelings out and off your chest; it's a release.

This is all you have control over. You will be successful if you accept that events of the past can't be changed, and that people outside of yourself can't be expected to respond the way you want them to. Thus, it's about expressing your feelings with no expectations.

STEP 16 *Expressing your feelings*

The energy associated with your feelings needs to be released, needs to be expressed. There are many ways to do this. As you visualize this person sitting opposite you, you may verbalize those feelings.

Again, the idea is to imagine the person really being there but recognize that he or she can't hear you, so there aren't any consequences. This allows you to be completely candid. If you are feeling angry, you can shout or even take up a pillow and smack the imaginary person sitting in front of you.

Even though this may seem strange, I encourage you to experiment and try different ways to express your feelings. You might also write a note. You can send the note, burn it, or tear it up.

STEP 17 *Accepting "what is"*

Again, remember that acceptance doesn't mean you like something; it simply is the recognition of reality. If you are unable or unwilling to accept, you will be stuck holding on to your feelings and probably becoming even more frustrated.

So, right now, if you have gotten all your feelings out, take a moment to recognize that what happened in the past can't be changed. Also, the person you are addressing is not going to change. Focus on your breathing.

STEP 18 *Any other feelings?*

Sometimes, at the moment of acceptance, you may for the first time experience a sense of loss.

The full impact of what you didn't have may come to the surface: loss of the childhood you would have wanted, loss of a loving parent you never had, loss of a safe and secure childhood, or loss of an accepting parent.

If this comes up, allow yourself any grieving that needs to take place. This is also part of the healing process!

STEP 19   *Continuing to focus on your breathing and letting go*

Make the decision right now that continuing to dwell on this issue can only hurt you without achieving anything. Note that this might bring up additional feelings of sadness and loss.

STEP 20   *Remembering joy*

Review your history and think back to a time when you experienced joy.

It could be over a period of time, or it might just be one brief moment.

Take yourself back to that time and picture yourself experiencing joy. Remember the moment in as much detail as possible. Where were you, who were you with, and what were you doing? Allow the energy of this positive experience to be felt right now, in this moment, in your body. Breathe into this feeling. With each release of old feelings, you might notice that your body is able to resonate and experience positive emotions just a little more fully.

A HEALTHY LOOK AT YOUR NEEDS

With your more significant unfinished emotional business, what makes it difficult to let go is that you are left with needs that were not met. Thus, either consciously or unconsciously, there is the drive to get these needs met. It is appropriate and necessary to deal with unmet needs. But it's easy to get stuck trying to get them met by someone incapable of doing that. It's like the guy standing under a lamppost at night looking at the ground. When asked, "What are you looking for?" he says, "I'm looking for my keys." "Well, where did you drop them?" the second person asks. And he points to a spot on the other side of the street. "Why are you looking here, if you dropped them over there?" "Because this is where the light is," replies the first man.

Yes, you need your keys (read: love, acceptance, attention, acknowledgment) and must get them. Don't keep looking where the keys won't be found! Also, be aware of the tendency to find people—new relationships—like the ones who were incapable of meeting your needs in the first place. The more you are able to address the emotional baggage you are carrying and let go, the more you are ready to find the right people to be in relationship with—people who are capable of meeting your needs. Take a moment to identify your unmet needs.

EXPERIENCING JOY, PLEASURE, AND PASSION

So many of the people I work with, when they frame the world, frame just half of it. How can you frame just half of the world? If your focus is to avoid anything negative, to hope that the worst doesn't happen and to be relieved when things turn out OK, then your frame only includes one-half of life's experiences.

If there were a vertical scale of life's events, the scale would have a baseline—a midpoint—and from this neutral place, the scale would go up into the positive and down into the negative. Concern for what might go wrong helps keep the focus on the lower half of this scale.

Recall the story of Jane, who always did well in her personal life and at work, getting "exceptional" ratings as an employee. But instead of rejoicing at doing so well, two other reactions were more prevalent: relief and pressure. There was relief that she got what she expected of herself (exceptional had become her norm), but she felt continuing pressure to keep doing just as well in the future. In fact, when we looked closely at this, she realized that when she got a great evaluation, after relief, her next thought was, "Now I will be expected to always do this well."

Many of you experience variations of this theme: anxiety that something might go wrong and relief when this doesn't happen. In addition, your anxiety and worry then get rewarded as you unconsciously believe: "I worried, and it turned out OK."

So, what is missing from this picture? Joy, excitement, and a full appreciation of your success. You are cutting off the top half of life's experiences—the joy and happiness of positive experiences. This focus is accentuated by the fear that too much joy or happiness might be followed by a crash, a turn of fortune. Of course, as pointed out previously, you also restrict the flow of energy by holding in your emotions.

Let's address all of these limiting factors in the next few steps on The Path. I am hoping you have followed the earlier steps of this chapter and addressed at least some of your emotional unfinished business. This, in itself, should release some of the tension in your body, allowing for a freer flow of energy. Let's take this further. The next few steps are particularly important for those who have not been experiencing a lot of joy in their lives. Follow steps twenty-one and twenty-two now.

STEP 21　*Rejoicing fully*

Visualize the full frame of life's experiences where the top half of this frame is positive, pleasurable, and happy. I now want you to focus solely on the top half of this frame. Give yourself permission to find something in your life to fully rejoice about.

What you identify doesn't have to be spectacular. This is an exercise where the goal is simply to practice your rejoicing ability.

Identify anything in your life that is positive. Fully immerse yourself in this memory or image and allow yourself to be joyful. If you are able, jump up and down, smile, laugh. As you do this, notice how good it feels. Breathe deeply and, as you do, allow your breath to carry the joy more deeply through your body. By doing this you are growing your capacity for joy.

STEP 22　*It's OK to experience happiness.*

Take a moment to check in with yourself and make sure you have no resistance to experiencing joy and happiness. We did this in a previous chapter, but let's do it again.

Say to yourself, "I deserve to experience joy and happiness just like everyone else." Make sure you are in resonance with this statement. Remember, this is what your healthy internal voice or internal parent would be saying. If you are having difficulty, it would be helpful to review the steps of the first pillar of resilience, relationship with self.

EMOTIONS AND THE FURTHER DEVELOPMENT OF CONFIDENCE AND SELF-EFFICACY

Full awareness of your feelings and the courage to go to difficult emotional places when necessary are the keys to emotional resilience and being on The Path. They are also the keys to developing confidence and self-efficacy. You are telling yourself, giving yourself the message, "I am willing to do what I need to truly help myself and to grow. If this means going to uncomfortable places, I will do it." This is the key to self-trust, the willingness to do what it takes to develop all aspects of yourself and then to realize you can count on yourself. This is going full circle from childhood, when you were dependent on others.

There are three ingredients to confidence: acceptance, the courage to do what's difficult, and appreciation of your efforts. Let's address them now in steps twenty-three, twenty-four, and twenty-five on The Path.

STEP 23 *Accepting and being true to yourself*

Life isn't about trying to be like someone else (although modeling some of your behavior on the optimal functioning of others is frequently a good idea). You can, at best, only be a copy of another person. But you can be a better you than anyone else; no one else is unique in quite the same way you are. Take a moment now to accept and even embrace who you are: Identify the parts of yourself that you love and accept your blemishes. Again, as noted previously, acceptance simply acknowledges "what is" without putting yourself down. It establishes a foundation from which to grow.

STEP 24   *The courage to do what's difficult*

If you have taken the earlier steps in this chapter on The Path, you have demonstrated courage. You have faced difficult feelings and actions. That's great. If you haven't, then now's the time to go back and select at least one person with whom to address your unfinished business. Recognize your courage to do the difficult. Each challenge you take requiring courage leaves you more equipped to embrace the next one.

STEP 25   *Appreciating your efforts*

Your growth doesn't take place in a straight line. The Path circles back on itself many times, and here is one example: There are many places and ways for you to appreciate yourself (as well as appreciating others). Every time you appreciate one of your efforts, you are emotionally nourishing yourself.

This contributes to your confidence, self-worth, and self-efficacy. And this, in turn, fosters greater resilience, as you (1) open to the nourishment, (2) reduce the uncertainty in your life by increasing your capacity to follow through, and (3) heighten your trust in yourself.

DON'T GET HIJACKED BY OTHERS' FEELINGS: NAVIGATING THE EMOTIONAL WATERS OF YOUR ENVIRONMENT

As you learn to take care of your own unfinished emotional business, you will find that you have fewer and fewer "buttons" that can be pushed. However, this doesn't take care of the emotionally wounded people you come into contact with. So, it's now important to address your management of the emotional energy surrounding you. At the top of this list is the impact on you, of the emotional turmoil of others, and your response to it. You want to be sensitive to the emotional pain of others but not allow it to become toxic to you.

You want to be aware of the emotional pitfalls that are present while not getting caught in them. Some examples include:

- Those who have not addressed their own unfinished business and thus carry around a backlog of feelings, such as anger. It might take very little to trigger these feelings toward you or anyone else. As noted in an earlier chapter, you might say it feels like "walking on eggshells" around these people.
- Those who project their own feelings onto others and therefore misinterpret your neutral or even unconscious actions as an intentional slight.
- Those who want to make you responsible for their feelings: "He should have known this would bother me."

There are many reasons a person you have a relationship with might be overly sensitive. We have discussed all of this in relationship to your own "stuff." You will encounter many people who are not on The Path, who are not interested or too scared to take a look at their own stuff. As a result, you may wind up in the crosshairs of their retribution or resentment.

You want to be sensitive to the emotions of others but not take responsibility for them. The challenge is being open to others while setting boundaries so you don't get hurt. Here are some steps to take in this process. Do steps twenty-six, twenty-seven, twenty-eight, and twenty-nine now.

STEP 26 *Noticing without reacting so you don't get drained by a bottomless pit*

The Buddhists would suggest having compassion toward these people. I would say that, first, you want to remind yourself that you are not responsible, and that getting upset will not make the other person's feelings go away; so why waste your energy with no benefit? Then go to a place of compassion. Remember, you don't have unlimited psychic energy.

STEP 27   *Don't jump to conclusions.*

Don't worry about what's going on with another person. Remind yourself that you are not a mind reader. You can't know what the other person really means. If you are wondering . . . ask.

STEP 28   *How to help regulate the emotions of others*

As you learned in pillar two, facial expressions cause reactions in your brain through the responses of mirror neurons. This is partly why we are unconsciously affected by our encounters. Use this to your own benefit.

Experiment with using a smile or a sympathetic or compassionate expression when engaged with someone who looks upset. Notice whether it softens their position, mellows them out, and disarms them.

STEP 29   *Don't let your emotions bleed onto others.*

The reverse is also true of you and your emotions. Yes, it's important to have a friend or relative with whom to vent and get out your feelings. But remember, there is an appropriate time and place for this.

It should not be done either indiscriminately or unconsciously. And you want to be careful not to make someone else responsible for your feelings.

REALLY FINISHING YOUR UNFINISHED BUSINESS

Using remote teaching methods, such as this book, I don't have the luxury of seeing your facial expression or using other methods of communication to detect whether you have fully addressed your unfinished business or have found a way to dismiss the process before reaching completion. But I do know how difficult the process is, and that there are many obstacles and pitfalls along the way.

Let's get one thing clear: You are not letting go of unfinished business to benefit someone else. It's not about letting him or her off the hook. You're doing it for yourself so you aren't still on the hook and held back. You are letting yourself off the hook of wasted energy and distraction. No one is feeling the effects of your holding on to feelings other than you (unless you are being passive-aggressive and trying to get the other person to feel guilty). Therefore, you owe it to yourself to accept, let go, and move on. This is what will help you be more present in life. The Path can only be found in the present moment. Do everything you can to let go of the past.

One last word of advice. Right now you are not looking for an intellectual "understanding." "Why did he treat me that way?" "Why didn't she show more affection?" Asking these questions is an additional way of holding on. You feel as though understanding will make everything right. The truth is, knowing that your father had a difficult childhood will be little consolation for how he treated you. When you were a child and received the emotional or physical harm, you were not able to minimize the hurt by any "understanding" of the events leading up to your treatment. Don't go there—it won't take away the hurts of the past. It will only distract you. Go to step thirty now.

STEP 30 *Another fearless accounting*

You are always welcome to return to your letting-go process. But right now, let's give it one more opportunity before moving on to pillar seven, presence.

Clear a few minutes of personal space and time. Carefully—and, I might add, ruthlessly—examine your relationships: Place each person in front of you and take time to "feel into" the connection.

Is there one or more person who stands out as still triggering feelings? Return to step twelve (and if necessary, even step three) and go through the process with this person or these people.

COMING FROM THE HEART

It is only fitting to bring your heart into this picture of emotional balance and mastery. In your personal encounters, you either come from the heart, or come from protecting the heart. The heart has, for centuries, been associated with one of our most cherished emotions: love. In fact, the heart is the most iconic symbol of love. The Buddha implored, "The way is not in the sky. The way is in the heart." And Helen Keller wrote, "The best and most beautiful things in the world cannot be seen or even touched—they must be felt with the heart."

I don't believe it's simply a metaphor to connect feelings with your heart. Carl Jung said, "Your vision will become clear only when you can look into your own heart. Who looks outside, dreams; who looks inside, awakes." He was referring to the emotional truth that lies inside your heart. That's where your emotions reside. When you have buried your feelings, you close your heart. To open your heart means to allow those feelings to be released and new ones to be received. Fear of experiencing our sadness, our losses, or reinjuring, keeps the heart closed. But as I've emphasized, it's impossible to be selective. As you close your heart to pain, you also close your heart to joy and love.

Remember the lesson from pillar four, physical balance and mastery. Coming from a place of love and gratitude fosters a coherent heart rate pattern, facilitating good health and healing. But when you hold negative emotions, the heart rate pattern becomes chaotic and harmful. Be fearless and have the courage to open and come from your heart. The rewards will be great. Here is a meditation you can practice to help in this process. Go to step thirty-one now.

STEP 31 *Cultivating an open heart*

Give yourself five to ten minutes to do this meditation. Create a safe space where you will not be interrupted.

Hold the intention to feel a sense of love and a connection with your heart. Turn your left hand facing up and place the pointer finger of your right hand on your pulse. This is your one-finger pulse exercise #1, as described in chapter ten. Take a moment to feel your pulse and make the connection with your heart. Establish a rhythmic breathing pattern, making each breath similar to the previous one.

If you are quiet enough, you can begin to notice the beating of your heart in your chest. In fact, imagine that when you breathe, you breathe the air directly into your heart.

To facilitate a sense of love and appreciation, identify a person in your life for whom you feel a sense of gratitude. Picture this person and hold him or her close to your heart. Remember, this is a developmental process. You are engaging in this meditative process to grow your sense of love and appreciation. I would even add that it's a way of growing your health. As you feel this sense of gratitude, imagine the feeling filling up your heart. Continue to breathe through your heart while focusing on feelings of love. Hold the intention of growing, and deepening, your feelings of love.

Try doing this meditation every day for seven days. Notice the effect it has on you. It's one more step you are placing on The Path.

Congratulations on a courageous and thoughtful engagement with this pillar of resilience and success. Remember to come from a place of acceptance. Appreciate what you have been able to accomplish and have compassion for the steps you were not able to do or had difficulty dealing with. I guarantee that every step you have taken has given you firmer footing on The Path.

SIGNPOST

- You have identified people who "push your buttons" and how you react.
- You have examined emotions that have been difficult for you to address.
- You have identified some of your fears in relationship to others.
- You have been working on coming from a place of acceptance—toward yourself and others.
- You have begun addressing your unfinished business with others.
- You have engaged in a process to experience your sense of joy and happiness.
- You have done the exercise of "acceptance, courage, and appreciation" to enhance your self-confidence and self-trust.
- You have learned ways of not reacting to the emotional upset of others.
- You have begun to cultivate the opening of your heart.

CHAPTER 13

PILLAR SEVEN
Presence: Gateway for The Path

I t is not possible to overestimate the power of presence in your ability to be resilient and successful. Life—all of life—takes place in the present, in this moment. It is a sacred place and space. It is where heaven is and where joy lives. You may shrink from it through fear, or leave it through numbing or distraction to avoid potential emotional pain, but you lose the joys of life as well. And, as I have explained, the emotional pain doesn't disappear, anyway; it just gets buried and becomes toxic!

In order for you to fully engage in life, to fully appreciate life and to function at your best, you must be as present, or in the moment, as possible. In fact, you can only affect or have an influence on your current life trajectory if you are present! We can say this another way: You must be present to shift from your old habitual patterns, your primitive Gestalt, to new, more successful ones. Being present is your gateway to The Path. As much sense as this makes, however, we spend most of our time somewhere else—in our heads or otherwise distracted, preoccupied by things from the past or worries about the future. Can you resonate with what I'm saying?

I remember a client, Gail, who was referred to me to treat symptoms resulting from an automobile accident. As I took her history, I grew increasingly incredulous as she reported a series of one automobile accident after another, for a total of six. Then came the kicker as she said, "None of these accidents was my fault." Was this some sort of weird streak of bad luck? Is it in fact possible to be involved in six automobile accidents and not be at fault? It reminded me of people I see stepping out into the crosswalk here in California, where the pedestrian has the right of way. They proceed to walk across the street, expecting traffic to stop—many don't even look to make sure an approaching car sees them! Well, it wouldn't be their fault if they got hit, but don't they have a responsibility to themselves to pay more attention?

As I began talking with and working with Gail, I noticed that she was not very present. She became distracted easily. If there was a pause in the conversation, she would quickly go into her head and into her thoughts. She was not tuned in to her environment. On occasion as she was leaving the office, she would brush into a wall, the table, or other objects in the environment, as if she didn't realize how close she was to them, that they were there; she wasn't aware of her relationship to objects around her. She was anywhere and everywhere but in the moment. She would be thinking and worrying about her children or her husband. Or she might be upset and self-critical about an interaction she had just had with me—or one from a few hours earlier. These were indications that those six accidents were probably because she wasn't present in the moment when they occurred, and thus she wasn't able to take evasive action.

Every one of Gail's thoughts or worries made her less able to function fully in the present. Being present is about "being in the moment" and not being preoccupied by things from the past or the future. It's also about minimizing automatic or habitual behaviors that foster unconsciousness and lack of awareness. Let me give you a few common examples of a lack of presence:

- You can be talking to someone yet not even notice what he or she is wearing.
- You can be speaking to a group of people and never look any of them in the eye.
- You can drive to work and not notice any of the details of the trip, including the streets you drove on—arriving without the awareness of the process of getting there.
- You can walk through a park and not notice the beauty all around you.
- You can be in a conversation with your wife, husband, or good friend and yet not really hear him or her because you are preoccupied with what you plan to say, some annoyance, or with a problem at work. As you were listening, something reminded you of a piece of unfinished business. And you shifted focus in an attempt to address this lingering problem. (Here is another example of the impact of our unfinished business.)
- You can leave a conversation but not really leave it as you hold on to a particularly unexplainable facial expression in the other person, thus interfering with your awareness of your environment and your next engagement.

These excursions from the moment interfere with awareness. Awareness is necessary for you to respond and adapt to changes in the environment and in your life. Awareness offers your body the opportunity to self-adjust and achieve balance. Awareness and presence are necessary ingredients for optimal third-stage neurogenesis—the growing of your brain cells. That puts you on The Path.

I have to add here that your interface with technology—be it phone, TV, or computer—has trained your brain to expect frequent shifts of focus. In your life you have gotten used to things changing rapidly, and you have learned to deal with the speed of change. The problem occurs when you want to stay focused on one thing and have a hard time doing it. In other words, you have been unconsciously trained to have a short span of attention.

This feeds into our tendency—developed through the evolutionary process—to orient to new stimuli. It was an important survival instinct for our hunter-gatherer ancestors, who needed to quickly recognize dangers in the wild. This is amplified by the reflex of going into our heads and memory banks to compare present situations with any similar past experiences that might indicate danger. Let's try a brief experiment to demonstrate how difficult it is to stay present. Do step one on The Path now.

STEP 1   *Assessing your presence*

I'd like you to focus on your breathing. Taking approximately ten seconds for a full breath, while counting four breaths and then starting from number one again. In other words, count your breaths like this: one, two, three, four, one, two, three, four, one, etc. Take a break and do this right now for just ninety seconds. No pressure or judgment, but let's check if you are able to go just ninety seconds following your breath and counting—or whether you get distracted before the end of this period. Use a watch with a second hand and begin the process right now. If you don't have a watch, do the exercise anyway, estimating the ninety seconds.

You might have noticed that you quickly got distracted from this process, losing track of the numbers. You may have noticed that you began getting tired or dizzy.

Perhaps you felt a bit uncomfortable and couldn't wait for the task to be completed. *Is this long enough?* you might have asked yourself. These are all indications of your difficulty in being present and staying focused. And it's true for most of us.

ADAPTATION LEADS TO LOSS OF PRESENCE

We know from biology that our sensing mechanisms adapt. If you're sitting next to someone wearing perfume, you may initially be distracted by the smell. New stimuli trigger an alerting response, which is sometimes referred to as an "orienting response," because you focus, tune in, or "orient" toward the new stimulus. But after a few minutes you may not even notice the smell.

These are demonstrations of our mind's ability and of our sensing mechanisms to adapt to non-changing stimulation. This ability to adapt is a good thing, but it can contribute to "brain laziness," or numbing to the environment—which leads you to ignore important signals you should pay attention to. It also leads to difficulty maintaining focus and presence. It can lead to the need for constantly new or changing stimuli to be able to stay focused. The key to optimal presence and being on The Path is to be flexible and able to notice changes but retain the ability to be focused when you need to attend.

CONTACT BOUNDARY: WHERE PRESENCE AND EXCITEMENT TAKE PLACE

The concept of the contact boundary was emphasized by Fritz Perls. He defined the contact boundary as that place where the "I" meets the environment. This can also refer to where the "I" meets one's internal environment—what you are noticing inside yourself as well as outside. It's at this contact boundary where true joy, excitement, growth, and perhaps nervousness occur.

If you are a person who is scared or fearful—and we all are to some degree—you will have a tendency to shrink from the contact boundary. We sometimes identify people like this as "shrinking violets." Perls would say that life happens at the contact boundary. He also noted, and I have found, that most people have great difficulty living right at that edge.

Pain and other uncomfortable experiences and feelings during your life motivate you to move away from the contact boundary. You might notice this as a tendency to "be in your head" or unconsciously jump to a different thought. When a conversation gets too close to your emotions, you might tell a joke or remember a story that takes you away from your discomfort—but also away from the moment. In psychology, we refer to this as a tendency to dissociate or deflect.

This takes us back to your old primitive Gestalt pattern. It's a normal reaction to move away from something painful. Think about how quickly your finger retracts from a hot stove. Even the cells in your body will constrict and close down when they detect a toxin in their vicinity. However, your tendency is the result of an old pattern that is no longer relevant. (It only continues to be relevant when you make inappropriate choices based on your early learning pattern, resulting in relationships similar to those of your childhood.)

To be at your best, to be most effective, and to be resilient you need to dwell as much as possible at the contact boundary. This is about embracing life and life's challenges. And here is where you will take your next steps onto The Path. Go to steps two and three now.

STEP 2 *Facilitating awareness in the present*

Review the one-finger pulse exercise: relaxation, growth, and resilience.

Use the exercise introduced in chapter ten, pillar four, to enhance presence and your ability to be in the moment; it will also enhance your resilience at the same time.

Turn your left hand palm up. Place your right index finger on your left wrist so that you can detect your pulse. Notice your pulse as you focus on a smooth and deep breathing pattern. Breathe in to the count of four and breathe out to the count of six, allowing your body to relax and let go as you exhale. Notice that your pulse quickens as you breathe in and slows as you breathe out.

Right now you are connecting with your internal environment. Feel your connection with your hands, your pulse, and your heart. Notice how present you are in this moment, and appreciate your effort to hang in there.

STEP 3 *Looking around and connecting with your environment as you continue to notice your breathing*

How is your nervous system functioning in this moment? Is it in fight-or-flight mode, more activated and "on guard" than necessary? If there is no real danger in the moment, use this opportunity to be present with your body, and allow yourself to turn down the activation of your nervous system by reminding yourself that you don't have to be on guard and that you are in a zone of safety.

Notice how present you are in this moment! Periodically, you can use this technique simply to bring yourself into the moment and, in addition, facilitate calmness.

WHERE IS YOUR CONTACT?

Right now you are focused on the material in this book, which guides your attention for the moment. When you finish this episode of reading, try to be aware of how you are making contact with your environment. First, are you able to stay in contact with the environment, or do you frequently go up into your head—into your thoughts? And if you do remain in contact, is it a clear or fuzzy contact? In other words, if you close your eyes, can you report what you just saw? Would you be able to say what color shirt the person you were talking to was wearing?

STRENGTHENING YOUR PRESENCE AND THE CONTACT CONTINUUM

Let me define the contact continuum, where being fully at the contact boundary is at one end of the continuum and being in your head deep in thought or worry is at the other end of the continuum. Understand that it's possible to be present while not really noticing. There is a gap between you and your environment. There is more of a vague experience of being present. Another way of saying this is that the quality of your contact is impaired. When this is happening, you are not fully taking in what is available through your five senses. Not everything is fully registering consciously. Thus, you are somewhere down the contact continuum. It's almost as if there is a veil between you and the world. This is also the case if you limit your awareness to only one of your sensory systems, such as visual. The goal is to be at the contact boundary as much as possible. The next exercise will help you become more aware and more present. This is a way to train yourself to dwell more at the contact boundary.

In this next process you will explore different ways of being present at the contact boundary. Your environment is complex, containing different shapes, objects, textures, colors, and people of all sizes. If you explore where the "I" meets the environment, there are many possibilities. You can observe with a wide focus, using a wide-angle approach, but without much detail. Or you can narrow your focus—looking at a specific object. You can view that object in detail or just its outline. You can observe something close to you in the environment or an object at a distance. We can break down the experience of the other senses in a similar manner. To strengthen your ability to focus, do steps four through nine now.

STEP 4   *Noticing how you make contact*

This exercise will help you begin to explore the contact boundary and discover where your own process gets stuck or perhaps is undeveloped. Right now, let's take in information about your environment. Next, close your eyes and report what you noticed.

How much of your environment did you take in? Did you recall information coming in from all five of your senses or just your visual perception?

Try it again: Notice your environment for about thirty seconds, then close your eyes and describe what you perceived.

Was this second experience different? If you only noticed the visual the first time, did you tune in to your other senses this time? Did you notice more details of your environment this second time?

STEP 5   *Look at what's in front of you.*

Now, take a closer look. Notice the objects in your view, but notice them in greater detail. And finally, take this one step further:

Pick an object and see if you can "place your eyeballs right on the surface of the object" as if there were no space in between. Actually see the texture, the color, and the shape of that object. This is a method for continually sharpening your awareness and gaining greater clarity.

It's a way of strengthening your presence. Whenever you have a moment, engage this process: look deeply into your environment.

STEP 6   *Let's do the same process, but now turn your awareness inward.*

Take a moment to notice your internal experience. Where is the focus of your attention? Is it in your head and in your thoughts?

Where do you begin to notice sensations and perhaps feelings in your body? Are you drawn to tension in a particular part of your body such as your neck or shoulders? Right now we can say that you are present with your internal experience. This is an important step in the awareness process. See if you can remember to do this a few times during the day today.

STEP 7   *Experiment with your attention*

Notice where in the environment you place your focus when you look up from this page. Do it now, for a moment. Notice if you are more tuned in to sights or sound; or perhaps you are eating and are more aware of taste and smells. Next, take a moment to look at a specific object. How many different ways can you see it? Can you see the entire object? If it's big, you might see just a part of it. But you might also focus in on a specific aspect of the object: its texture, its shape, or its color.

STEP 8 *Next, experiment with varying your focus*

First take a wide-angle view of your environment, seeing the big picture. Notice as you do this that most of your visual field is diffuse, meaning it's difficult to see anything in detail. Now, continue with this same wide view. But at the same time, notice the detail in one object.

This perceptual challenge improves brain function and enhances awareness. You can extend this process by shifting to other objects in your visual field and then also by bringing in your other senses.

STEP 9 *Synesthesia, experiencing an integration of your senses*

This last way of engaging your senses is referred to as synesthesia. This is where you see a sound, or experience a color along with a sound. It is where the stimulation of one sensory pathway, such as sight, activates a different sensory pathway, such as smell or taste. At some point in your day today, experiment with the integration of your different senses. Try to experience an image as you listen to a sound, such as music. Can you taste an odor?

MINDFULNESS TRAINING TO FACILITATE CONTACT AND A CALM FOCUS

Ancient traditions, such as Buddhism and other spiritual approaches, have emphasized the active cultivation of awareness and conscious attention. This process has been advanced through the contemporary practice of mindfulness. Attention and awareness are features of normal functioning, but as you are learning, many factors impair our ability to be present. Mindfulness is another approach that will improve your ability to be present and stay at the contact boundary. It can also improve your ability to develop a calm focus, your new twenty-first-century stress response.

Most of the time we are walking around half-asleep. This is, as I've been saying, when we are on automatic and following our old patterns and habits and are barely aware of our surroundings or what we are doing. This is in contrast to having heightened states of clarity and sensitivity. Our history of trauma, pain, and other emotional hurts results in fears and judgments that cause us to shrink from the contact boundary. Mindfulness is the process of being aware and noticing without judgment—of being present without reacting. It's like being a neutral observer of your life—in the moment. The more you can remove emotional reactivity, the greater your presence will be.

Mindfulness of the ancient type or of the more current form has been shown to enhance self-regulation and well-being. Scientific research has validated the positive emotional and physical benefits from employing this technique. Go to step ten on The Path now. This is also a good time to review and reinforce the training from your second, one-finger pulse exercise. Go to steps eleven and twelve on The Path to continue this training.

STEP 10   *Practicing one minute of mindfulness*

Give yourself one minute right now to activate positive and calming brain circuits. Do this by simply noticing where your focus goes, without making any judgments about it. It might go to what you are observing in your environment, and then you might have thoughts about future plans, and then you might notice a physical sensation. Allow each of these awarenesses to be present without judgment, almost like a movie playing before you. Do this right now for sixty seconds. As a mindfulness practice, you can enhance it with the one-finger pulse exercise #1. When you are done, notice how you feel. Doing this exercise on a regular basis has been shown to improve happiness and well-being. Try extending your periods of mindfulness.

STEP 11 *Achieving calm focus*

Two-finger pulse exercise

Right now, imagine a stressful situation in your life. Visualize it, and notice how it activates your body. To do this, follow the two-finger pulse exercise.

This will indicate that you are in a stressful situation and that you want to go into a calm, focused state. Notice your pulse as you breathe in to the count of four and out to the count of six. In this exercise, say to yourself, "I want to be focused and alert to handle the stress, but at the same time, I can stay calm. I can achieve just as much, if not more, than if I'm tense and stressed."

Then go into your optimal breathing pattern as you imagine engaging with the stressful situation. This is a process you can engage in on a regular basis to retrain and literally reengineer your stress response and help you remain calmer under stress.

STEP 12 *Reviewing the two techniques*

Relaxation, growth, and resilience:

1. When you determine there isn't any real danger, place your index finger on your left wrist pulse, and then, as you feel it, breathe slowly, let go, and relax deeply.

Redesigning your fight-or-flight response:

2. Place your middle and index fingers on your right wrist pulse when there is a real concern, danger, or pressure. Remind yourself that you can achieve more with a calm focus. Then go into your calm breathing pattern while staying focused on addressing the source of your stress.

CHOICE AND THIRD-STAGE NEUROGENESIS

For optimal development and personal growth—at the heart of resilience and success—you have to be able to make choices. As discussed previously, neurogenesis will take place even if you are acting out of habit and old patterns, but the new nerve growth will only reinforce the same tired ways of doing things. Each moment you are present you give yourself the opportunity to make new decisions, to choose a new direction that puts you on The Path. When this happens, you are triggering more effective new nerve growth and rewiring your brain circuitry to solidify these new choices. I have called this "third-stage neurogenesis."

Every moment you are present, you have the choice to wake up, to choose to let go of physical tension instead of going along with familiar muscle tensing; to think differently—more positively instead of negatively or critically; to feel differently—experiencing feelings instead of ignoring them. And the effect is cumulative. Do steps thirteen and fourteen now.

STEP 13 *Practicing a quick technique to become present*

The easiest way to bring yourself into the present moment is through your five senses. Let's do this right now.

Take a moment to notice what you are seeing, hearing, smelling, tasting, and touching. As you connect with information coming in through your five senses, you are immediately brought right into the present moment. This is the only place you can sense, and this is a great technique to bring yourself into the present at any time.

STEP 14 *Creating opportunities for positive choices using "portals"*

This is an exercise I learned through my study of George Gurdjieff, who taught ways of awakening one's consciousness. For the rest of this day, every time you walk through a portal—a door or an entryway—use this cue to bring yourself to the present moment, to "remember yourself."

Be conscious of your surroundings. Ask, "What is my intention in this moment?" Sometimes it might be a mundane activity such as washing your hands, but at other times, it might cause you to think more clearly about an old behavior—such as being critical, having a candy bar, or procrastinating. It might cause you to stop and ask yourself whether your next activity is important in moving you toward your goals. Use any portal to wake up in the moment and make optimal choices!

OPTIMAL PRESENCE

Optimal presence begins to incorporate some of the lessons from the first six pillars of resilience and success. For example, you want to be present in the moment while coming from a place of acceptance toward yourself as opposed to being judgmental or critical. It also means having a positive attitude about what you are experiencing and not being negative. Your presence, your focus in the moment, is like a laser directing your attention and experience straight to your brain. The quality of your presence will determine which brain circuits get activated and thus reinforced. Each time you are present in an accepting and positive way, you are building resilient and successful brain pathways. When you combine presence with intention, you consciously ignite neuroplasticity.

GRATITUDE

We tend to bring our attention to things that need to be fixed or changed. Our radar picks up the dangers, problems, and what's wrong. Yet there is much to be grateful for in our lives. The song "The Best Things in Life Are Free" has some truth to it. In his book, *Thanks! How the New Science of Gratitude Can Make You Happier*, Robert Emmons shares his research that demonstrates how a focus on gratitude in your life can lead to improved emotional and physical health. And

Dr. Rollin McCraty of the HeartMath Institute (IHM) has shown that feeling gratitude enhances coherent heart rate patterns. These patterns facilitate the alignment of many biological rhythms. Cathy Holt of IHM says the coherent patterns that arise from a state of gratitude can "enhance our immune response, problem solving and intuition, and balance our nervous system."

No matter what is going on in your life, there are many things to be grateful for. You can be grateful that you awoke this morning and that when you opened your eyes you saw beautiful colors. You can look up at the sky and appreciate the uniqueness of the cloud formations and how they continuously change into different and complex patterns. You can appreciate the level of health that you do have. You can hold a place of gratitude for the variety of foods you eat. Above all, it's important to acknowledge and appreciate those in your life who are there for you, support you, and love you. What can you be grateful for? Do step fifteen now.

STEP 15 | *Exercising your gratitude muscle*

Think about someone in your life for whom you have gratitude. Do this in conjunction with your one-finger pulse exercise #1 (pointer finger on pulse). Take a moment to hold him or her in your heart and feel appreciation. Breathe, and as you do, notice how good this makes you feel. Notice your pulse and imagine it going into a coherent and rhythmic pattern. When you go to sleep this evening, take a moment to identify things in your life that you are grateful for. Tomorrow morning, when you awaken, start your day with a moment of gratitude and appreciation. From now on in your life, take time each day—including morning and evening—to be grateful and hold this place of gratitude.

As you follow this step on The Path, make note of how it makes you more positive and happier. Also, notice how it helps you be more in the present.

FOSTERING AN ACTIVE PARTICIPATION IN LIFE AND GROWTH—OVERCOMING HELPLESSNESS

Your primitive Gestalt pattern contributes to an underlying passivity in the development of your sense of self. In fact, I might even refer to this as learned helplessness, where who you are is set by your childhood story. You might notice this in your self-comments, such as, "I can't do this," "That's not me," or in the ceiling that has been unconsciously placed over you—your unspoken limitations.

Psychologists discovered learned helplessness through research that repeatedly subjected animals to an adverse stimulus, such as shock, that they could not escape. Eventually the animals stopped trying to avoid the pain, giving up and acting helpless to change the situation. When this happens, even when the opportunity to escape is subsequently presented, the learned helplessness interferes with taking action.

There are many ways in which, as children, we are limited in our ability to change uncomfortable situations. This contributes to a lack of empowerment—or learned helplessness. When we become adults, learned helplessness turns into a passive attitude toward making changes in who you are and what you can accomplish. Think of your primitive Gestalts as setting a boundary that establishes who you think you are and what is within your power. This boundary then sets a limit on your growth, what I've called first and second levels of neurogenesis. Breaking this pattern is one of the most important steps in your ability to become resilient and successful. So here are the two attitudes you can take when you meet with frustration, an obstacle, or repeated failure at change:

1. You can get discouraged as you keep trying to make a change and the same things keep occurring. You keep trying, but the negative voice has gotten to you. The change seems almost impossible. The result is that you become unsure whether you will ever be able to achieve your goal, or get beyond the level you have achieved. When this happens, the voice of the

primitive Gestalt has won—and it knows it. This is also a part of a "fixed mindset."

2. When you face your shortcomings as you realize you again were unconscious and made the same mistake, or repeated an action in the same ineffective manner, you reaffirm your intention and your commitment to do whatever it takes to learn, grow, and be more effective. You declare to yourself, "I won't give up until I get it right" and "I will no longer use excuses when I'm not successful." With this attitude, you are telling yourself that you will never give up, no matter what, until you achieve success! This is part of a healthy "growth mindset."

When you take this second attitude with conviction—"no matter what, I won't give up"—you are putting the old voice on notice. You decide you are not going to be defined anymore by your old story. When you do this, when you hold this intention, real change and growth become possible. The more you are able to be present and make this choice, the more you have the potential to say, "I'm going to establish a new story," "I'm going to focus on new possibilities for myself," and thus you are on The Path. This fosters third-level brain cell regeneration, growth, and healthy development. This is resilience! Can you say this now: "No matter what, I won't give up." Johann Wolfgang von Goethe put it this way: "The moment one definitely commits oneself, then Providence moves too." Go to step sixteen.

STEP 16 | *Becoming a more active participant in your life—an affirmation*

Right now create an affirmation that says you are taking a more active and positive role in how you live your life. Here are a couple of examples: "It's up to me to determine the results I get in life." "I will do whatever I need in order to develop positive life patterns. This will result in me being happier, healthier, and more successful." "I will no longer be defined by my story and the ways I have done things in the past."

DEVELOPING A STRONG "WILL"

People talk about having a strong will as if it is something you are born with. In fact, will is a quality to be developed. When you take a stand, when you fight on in the face of frustration, fear, uncertainty, or even defeat, you are developing a strong will. This process is advanced even in situations in which you don't achieve your ultimate goal. Your will is strengthened every time you have the courage to act in the face of fear or uncertainty. Go to step seventeen now.

STEP 17   *Strengthening your will*

Identify a current struggle, procrastination, or even a perceived failure you are experiencing. What is your fear? How can you call on your healthy internal parent to support you taking a step anyway? Take a moment to recommit to doing what it takes to achieve success. What action do you need to take? Schedule this action now.

THE SOLIDITY OF YOUR CENTER—KNOWING WHERE YOU STAND!

You have many different "I"s: the "I" connected with accomplishment, the "I" connected to relationships, the "I" that's devoted to someone or something, etc. Presence is the opportunity to bring all of these "I"s together under one roof. Usually, these "I"s pull you in different directions—with different and usually unconscious goals. In previous chapters I referred to this as resulting from your unfinished business and unmet needs. But it's also due to old rules and rules handed down that no longer serve you.

There is no actual location for your psychological center. Let me help you visualize how your center works. Imagine walking on a wooden plank that's elevated high above the ground. Let's say this piece of wood is about five feet wide. Now let's say that at both ends, where the board rests on solid platforms, the wood narrows to only two feet, so that as you place your weight more to the sides of the plank, the shakier and more precarious the plank gets. Under these circumstances, it is best to be in the center, where you will experience the greatest solidness and stability.

For the same reason, your psychological center is where you are the most solid and grounded. Your center should be a source of strength. The center is the place inside from which you trust yourself. When you continue living by the rules of others and the outmoded lessons from your childhood, the less you know your own center—and the less you can trust yourself. If you are allowing yourself to be guided by the judgments of others, there is always uncertainty. It's as if you are living on the sides of the plank, where it's shaky, but you're wondering why you don't feel solid. Finding and standing on your center is about coming to your own conclusions about what's true for you and taking a stand (and risk) based on a thoughtful and unemotional determination. Finding your center is also about owning and standing on your abilities, rather than doubting them, thus contributing to the stability of what you are standing on.

The more you take responsibility for your positions in life, the more trust you have in yourself and the more you know where you stand. This puts you smack-dab in the middle of that plank. This fosters confidence and self-trust. It also helps bring all your "I"s together within your presence. The more you are in the present and are true to yourself, the more you can trust yourself. The more you decide and declare what's true for you—as opposed to living by the rules set up by your parents and others—the more you can trust yourself. A strong center is based on this self-trust! The stronger this center, the greater your self-confidence and the less dependent you are. When you then connect with others it will be from a place of strength, which also results in greater presence and resilience. This is truly walking on The Path. Do steps eighteen, nineteen, and twenty now.

STEP 18   *What can you stand on?*

Identify a few things that you trust about yourself. It might be your reliability or your persistence. It might be a technical ability or your facility with numbers. It might be how easily you make friends.

STEP 19   *What rules can you finally make that are your own?*

Maybe you have been prejudiced by default, taking on the bias of your parents or your culture. It's now time to determine your own position and where you stand on this or some other rule you may be outgrowing. For example, you can make a new rule that it's OK to feel and express your feelings. Perhaps you might make a new rule that it's OK to be spontaneous. Identify a new rule and a stand you can take now.

STEP 20   *"I am here." This is a declaration of your presence.*

Make this statement to yourself as you reaffirm your belief in yourself. Johann Wolfgang von Goethe said, "Magic is believing in yourself. If you can do that, you can make anything happen."

PROJECTING PRESENCE

Up to now, I've been discussing presence from a receiving perspective. Awareness, paying attention, noticing, and focus are all about what is coming in through your senses. In this manner you have been aware of your internal and external environments, what we might refer to as input. This is what people typically mean when they refer to presence. But I want to talk about what I consider the other side of presence, the projecting side: what you project out into the world. What is your impact on others? The last two sections on "will" and your center have led up to this discussion.

I like to think of presence as a two-way street. In addition to the input component, there is also an output or projecting side. This is the energy you send out into your environment and to others. It's about the energy you bring to individual moments of your life. Remember the lessons of earlier chapters, in which I indicated that sophisticated instruments can detect your heartbeat in the brain waves of people standing close to you? This is a concrete indication of the power of your "presence," the unspoken and usually unconscious impact you have on other people.

We often encounter individuals we want to be close to. These people have charisma, an attracting force about them. Many people in the public eye fit this category. For example, the energy that former president Bill Clinton projects is powerful and legendary. But you don't have to be a superstar to project positive energy and to benefit from this approach. Altruism is defined as the principle or practice of unselfish concern for or devotion to the welfare of others. I would suggest that when you are thinking of others, and spreading warmth and love, it will reflect back to you in spades. Others will feel good around you, want to be with you, and want you to succeed. When you are on The Path, you automatically gravitate to these people—and you are in the process of becoming one of these people.

There are also people whom you want to get as far away from as possible. These people project a very different kind of energy. When you are in their presence, you might immediately feel some discomfort. It may be a feeling that you are being judged. Or the other person might simply appear unhappy or just slightly annoyed or bored. The feeling is not welcoming.

These people typically have not addressed or resolved their own unfinished business and therefore carry around emotional baggage that seeps out in their "presence." Unresolved anger, for example, affects heart rate, creating a chaotic pattern. Love affects heart rate in an entirely different way, creating greater harmony or coherence. Some people can cause tension in others simply by walking into a room.

Unfortunately, if you grew up with this type of person, say your mother or father, you will experience conflict: The part of you still experiencing unmet needs will be attracted, while the part of you wanting to be healthy will want to stay away from this person. As I discussed in pillar two, your relationship with others, it's important for your emotional health to be discriminating and hang out with people who have a positive presence. These are the only people truly capable of meeting your needs.

In everyday life, each of you has a public presence and image. This is a part of what's referred to as "emotional intelligence." Your actions and behavior are certainly part of this image, but your presence, or how people experience you when they are in your presence, is a major factor. Your presence is an important part of resilience and success. A positive presence can break down barriers and predispose others to be on your side and want to help you. We can say that you thus align the energies and forces surrounding you in your favor. In other words, projecting a positive presence puts you on The Path. Projecting a negative presence will have the opposite effect and create resistance—friction—along your path, the same way you react to a person who projects negativity.

YOUR PUBLIC IMAGE

Cary Grant, a debonair actor who projected tremendous confidence, was once asked about his image. To the surprise of the interviewer, Grant said that he consciously cultivated that image. He decided how he wanted others to perceive him and adopted this image until it became natural to him.

I'm aware that this notion of acting "as if" may appear contradictory to previous messages about integrity: that is, aligning your internal world (what you believe about yourself) with what you project out to the world. Here is the difference. If you hold up a model of your goal, how you want to become, and strive toward becoming this, there is no lack of integrity. If you work on projecting a positive, confident self as you strive to be on The Path, there is no discrepancy. You are working on the same goals on different levels. You might also object to the perceived artificiality of a public image in this age of image "makers." However, the reality is that we all have a public image. Be intentional about yours. It's time to do steps twenty-one through twenty-four on The Path.

STEP 21 · *Identifying someone with a positive presence*

Take a moment to identify someone in your life whom you like being with. Picture this person in your presence right now. Notice how you feel when you are with him or her. What are the qualities of this person that attract you? Is it her smile? His positivity? Perhaps it's the individual's obvious interest in you and your life? You might be attracted to her "take charge" attitude in life. Stay with the image of this person and enjoy the feeling for a few more moments, as well as noticing the qualities you are appreciating.

STEP 22 · *What is your presence—the energy you project?*

It's time to engage in an honest assessment of your own presence—the energy you project. Reflect on your interactions with others, among them family, friends, and business associates.

As you review and remember these encounters, what do you notice about your energy? Are you inviting or guarded? Is your energy positive or negative? Open or constricted? Whatever it is that you notice, are you satisfied with what you perceive or with the feedback you receive? Is it getting you the results you want?

STEP 23 · *What shift in your presence do you want to make?*

Identify some aspect that you would like to improve. It might be showing greater interest in the other person. It might be the projection of a greater sense of confidence or of joy in your life. You might simply intend to have a more upright posture or put a smile on your face when you greet others. Make some commitment to adjust your presence right now and make sure you follow through. Write it down on one of your affirmation cards so you won't forget.

STEP 24 *Projecting a positive "self"*

What qualities do you appreciate about yourself? How can you project them out into the world and toward the people you make contact with?

Let's use the concept of "portals," or entryways again, as a signal, a cue to remember yourself. Today, use this cue to strengthen the presence you project out into your world. Each time you walk through a portal, either to meet a person, a group of people, or simply to walk out into the world, think about your positive qualities and allow them to fully occupy the space within you. Then straighten your posture, breathe, smile, imagine projecting positive energy, and make eye contact with whomever you greet.

HOMEOSTASIS AND NOTICING YOUR NEEDS

Sometimes we forget how perfectly our bodies are designed. Homeostasis is our body's built-in intention and goal always to remain in balance. Your nervous system continually monitors thousands of biological processes, from blood pressure and blood sugar levels to hydrochloric acid levels in your stomach. Any time one of these systems is out of balance, your body detects it and sends a signal to make an adjustment to restore balance. Thus a message may get sent to dilate blood vessels to lower blood pressure or for the kidneys to release water to adjust blood sugar levels. Most of these adjustments occur without you noticing them.

But there are also systems in your body that are not handled automatically. These require your awareness and the recognition that a need has arisen. Hunger, for example, requires an awareness of a physiological discomfort, followed by efforts to acquire and ingest food. The same is true for the recognition of your emotional needs. One of the most important goals of being present is the ability to notice these needs so you can take the necessary actions to meet the need. The more present you are able to be, the more you will notice needs. We can say this another way: you will allow a need to emerge as a figure that stands out from the background. Do step twenty-five now.

STEP 25 *Noticing your needs*

Take a moment to tune in to your body and your environment. Breathe and let go. Can you detect a need, either emotional or physical? Are you thirsty? When was the last time you had a glass of water? Are you aware of needing emotional support or the caring or acknowledgment of another person? Perhaps you just became aware of feeling annoyed at a particular person and need to find a way to release this feeling.

BEING PRESENT IS YOUR RESPONSIBILITY

I want to conclude this chapter with an idea that summarizes the subject of presence: responsibility. At the heart of presence and, thus, at the heart of being on The Path is you being responsible for the quality, success, and happiness of your life. Take this responsibility as seriously as anything else you ever do. Incorporate this into your commitment and intention to be successful and resilient and to be on The Path. To ensure this happens, incorporate into your daily affirmations a statement about practicing one of the presence exercises of this chapter on a daily basis. And include an affirmation about being responsible or taking responsibility for your life, your resilience, and your success.

I want to appreciate you for getting to this point on The Path.

SIGNPOST

- You have continued to use the two versions of the one-finger pulse exercise for greater presence.
- You have engaged in exercises to strengthen your ability to be at the contact boundary.
- You have explored different ways of noticing and being aware.
- You have begun using the technique of portals.
- You have practiced the five-senses exercise.
- You have practiced mindfulness, noticing without judgment.
- You are exercising your gratitude muscle.
- You are shifting from being a passive observer to becoming a more active participant in your life.
- You are learning what you stand for and locating your center, in order to say, "I am here."
- You are projecting positive energy out into your world.
- You are getting more in touch with your needs so they can be met.

CHAPTER 14

PILLAR EIGHT
Flexibility

As mentioned previously, I had the good fortune to get to know neuroscience pioneer Donald Hebb when I was an assistant professor at McGill University in Montreal. Don would go back to his native Hebbville, Nova Scotia, during the summers. His home was right on the ocean. The first time I visited, he took me out on his sailboat. I was a bit wary, as he was over seventy at the time, and we were going out into the Atlantic. I said, "I can help. I've sailed before." As if to appease me, he said, "Good," with a slight smile on his face. When we got to his boat, I found it to be an odd shape, coming to a point at the front and back—bow and stern, respectively—of the craft. When I asked him about it, he said, "The design is forgiving of slowness and mistakes. So I figure I bought myself an extra five years of sailing." Looking back, this was a great example of flexibility.

Many years ago, the United States experienced the "British invasion," when the Beatles came across the "pond" to excite fans and were followed by a wave of imitators. Today there is a new invasion, and this time it's from India. It's the "yoga invasion." More than fifty million people in this country are now doing yoga on a regular basis! Much of the benefit that accrues from yoga practice stems from its enhancement of physical flexibility and range of motion. It is also a model for the benefits of flexibility as the eighth pillar of resilience and success, which includes reducing resistance, bending without breaking, and ongoing rejuvenation.

Flexibility is also the ability to adapt—to learn from new experiences and new information and not be stuck in outmoded ways of doing or thinking. It is the ability to be open, to see different perspectives, to put yourself in other people's shoes, and to learn from varied sources. This frequently involves letting go of the old. If you're flexible, you can adjust and become comfortable with new, different, and unexpected circumstances, rather than let these situations create distress. As the saying goes, you want to "turn lemons into lemonade." Flexibility is the ability to shift goals for easier success. As author Patricia Ryan Madson said, "If something is not to your liking, change your liking."

Flexibility is interacting with the environment without being restricted by rigid beliefs of how you should respond. Any belief system becomes a prison if one holds to it too firmly.

Your primitive Gestalt pattern imprinted during childhood—the pattern we have been working on recognizing and letting go of—contributes to your loss of flexibility. It's as if a boundary is established: What's inside is you; what is outside is not you, so don't go there. Such a fixed, closed boundary inhibits growth. You unconsciously experience this countless times each day. As soon as you get close to your boundary or there is a chance you might step over it, you begin to feel uncomfortable. This may occur in response to a compliment, where the discomfort you feel interferes with letting it in. You may have experienced this discomfort when you first began doing one of the relaxation exercises in this book. As you started to become calm, feelings began to bubble up that triggered the discomfort, and you may have stopped the process. Or you may have completely resisted doing a relaxation exercise because, again, it's outside your experience and thus not what you do.

Numerous psychological experiments have demonstrated that personal bias determines how and what you perceive. You are more likely to see what it is you are expecting to see and miss much of the environment in the process. In addition, you are more likely to notice the negative, the potential dangers, rather than what's positive and calming. This tendency limits new learning and new growth. It also occurs, as discussed previously, when your brain falls into a rut.

Flexibility, in my model of resilience, is at the heart of health. It reflects a key ingredient of learning: dancing with experience without being constrained by fear or prejudgment about how that experience should be or jumping to conclusions about how it is. In this way, it's possible to be fully open to what the experience has to offer as it unfolds.

Not only is the world changing, but the pace of change keeps speeding up. There is an exponential growth in knowledge and in the amount of information available. It's more important than ever to be flexible and adapt to these changes. Charles Darwin, the English naturalist and geologist, said: "It is not the strongest or the most intelligent who will survive but those who can best manage change." Yet, as Ken Wilber noted, "Most of us are only willing to call five percent of our present information into question at any one point." How much of your behavior and thinking are you willing to question?

STALKING YOUR PATTERN; RIGIDNESS OF YOUR BELIEFS

Think of a way in which you are limited by your thinking and fixed beliefs.

This might be your thinking about yourself, such as "I'm not good enough," "I can't do it," or some other way that you place a ceiling over yourself. It might be your beliefs about the world and others, such as "People will judge me, and that's scary," or "It's not all right to make a mistake, so I better not try to achieve this goal."

Think about your own primitive Gestalt pattern and how your beliefs limit you. Perhaps you don't believe you can really follow through and finish something. Perhaps you are unsure of your ability to commit or to be fully present, based on past experience. Possibly you need to wait for someone else to validate an idea before you believe it for yourself.

Perhaps, as you get close to completing a project, you get distracted or become anxious and miss an opportunity for success.

These are all examples of your lifelong habitual patterns and ways that you think about yourself and the world that interfere with your ability to be flexible, to try new approaches, to consider new ideas. And to grow into a more complete version of yourself. Your pattern is with you all the time and guides your thinking and behavior. It's important to be aware of how you are influenced by these fixed beliefs.

This awareness is facilitated by what I'm referring to as "stalking your pattern." Picture a tiger in the wild, hunting for food. It will get into a crouch as it moves intentionally and smoothly, keeping a low profile to avoid being seen. The tiger is stalking its prey. It's paying close attention, keeping the prey in sight. Or the animal might not yet have seen its prey but is using its other senses of smell and hearing to pick up traces of its prey. During this process it's very focused on the task and nothing can distract it.

I want you to think of your pattern as your prey. Since it's always a part of you, it is continually displaying itself. In fact, you might even notice the presence of your pattern in how you approach learning about The Path. You might be hard on yourself when you forget to do a relaxation exercise. Or, you might think of change as being very difficult and thus create resistance to the process.

Your pattern, your primitive Gestalt, can be considered what is inside the boundary of who you are and what you do. Outside of this boundary would therefore be everything you think of as "not you." It consists of beliefs, behaviors, and qualities. For example, dancing might be outside your boundary, and even positive expectations might be outside your boundary. Right now, go to steps one through seven on The Path.

STEP 1 *Stalking your pattern*

Beginning today, pick out aspects of your pattern in your behaviors and thinking: stalk your pattern.

STEP 2 *Defining your boundaries*

Visualize a circle that surrounds who you are; leave what you are not outside the circle. Identify a few of the things outside your circle, such as being healthy, smart, funny, successful, or confident.

Can you think of where this holds you back, interferes with your self-interest, or contributes to your procrastination?

STEP 3 *Identifying what's inside the circle of who you are*

Let's do this in two parts: first, those aspects of yourself that are assets, that you appreciate; second, those parts you consider a liability.

For example, an asset might be your ability to solve problems, while a liability might be your fear or procrastination. An asset might be your likability; a liability might be your unreliability or difficulty following through, which leads to not trusting yourself.

STEP 4 *What assets lie inside your circle?*

Be as comprehensive as possible. Facilitate this process by thinking of someone who loves you. What would they say are your assets, those things that are inside your circle?

STEP 5 *What liabilities lie inside your circle?*

Try to list these weaknesses without adding any commentary or self-abuse. Be as neutral as possible.

STEP 6   *Listing what's outside the circle*

These are qualities or abilities you want. You might want to be someone who keeps his or her commitments. You might want to own your successes and accept compliments gracefully.

STEP 7   *Flexing your boundary*

For a moment, imagine that this boundary is flexible. It has the ability to flex outward to expand and, by doing so, incorporate something that is outside. This might be the ability to complete what you start. Right now, whether it's this or something else you identify, imagine that it's suddenly within your boundary of who you are.

If you can hold this image and keep returning to it, you will instigate new nerve connections, as you mentally expand your boundary. This is putting you on The Path toward making it a reality.

BRAIN, BEHAVIOR, AND FLEXIBILITY

What's most familiar, what gets rewarded, gets wired into your brain networks. Again, "What fires together, wires together." If we examine what happens in the brain during the process of learning, we discover that new connections are made between neurons, and new brain circuits are created. Even new brain structures are created, such as synaptic nodes: little protrusions on a neuron that increase communication between it and other neurons. When new, learned behavior is repeated, the neurons in these new circuits will fire and thus get wired through this building-and-strengthened process, making the behaviors more and more likely to be repeated and further strengthened.

The more a brain circuit—which represents learned behavior—is strengthened, the more your brain wants to go down these familiar pathways. That's OK. In fact, it's a good thing. It can improve performance and encourage faster responses. But when you want to be open to new ideas and more optimal ways of doing and thinking, it is important for your brain to be flexible, so it can shift and go into new patterns for new learning.

In other words, the irony is that the more a learned pattern is strengthened, the more the brain falls into a rut in which these patterns become the default behaviors, making new or different behaviors—new learning—less likely. And when these patterns are created in childhood during survival learning, they form your primitive Gestalt. The key to staying vital and being open to new ideas and new ways of being is flexibility. In fact, this might be a good definition of creativity.

Adaptability and being able to learn from new experiences is the key to healthy growth and optimal functioning. The loss of flexibility or adaptability speeds up the aging process.

What we want to achieve is the perfect balance between following the healthy lessons we've already learned and being open to new lessons. It's a good thing if the lessons you are learning become positive habits. Do step eight on The Path now.

STEP 8 *Allow yourself to be awkward*

Let's begin with some non-threatening ways of behaving differently in order to integrate the left and right sides of your brain. For the rest of today, try using your non-dominant hand to perform routine and familiar tasks such as eating or brushing your hair or teeth. As you do this, notice how it feels, notice any awkwardness and any judgments you make.

Try doing this from a place of adventure and curiosity. It's a safe way to experience the awkwardness of new behavior. And finally, if you do this for any length of time, notice what happens. Do you begin to get impatient because everything takes longer? Or do you begin to notice that you feel less awkward, or that it gets easier?

Let's now use this notion of brain flexibility and integration of the two sides of your brain to address an uncomfortable feeling. Do steps nine and ten now.

STEP 9   *Identify an uncomfortable situation*

Think of a situation, with a place or a person, where you begin to have an uncomfortable or anxious feeling or begin to feel tense. It may occur as you enter a room filled with people, or it may happen when you are alone. It might happen as you start to do a difficult task.

Identify what the discomfort is about. Perhaps you can trace it to an old interaction or an ongoing experience from childhood in which you were criticized or felt unprotected. Talk to yourself about this discomfort and where it comes from. Be as specific as possible.

By talking to yourself about a feeling, you are automatically connecting the two sides of your brain: the feeling side, and the more cognitive and verbal side. Let's take this one step further.

STEP 10   *Shift your perspective*

If this situation were happening to someone you care for (think of a specific person), what would you tell him or her? How would you reassure that individual? Now, encourage your own flexibility by using this same approach to reassure yourself. Notice whether this process helps lower your discomfort.

In order to help you become more open to new ways of being in the world and new ways of seeing yourself, it's important to further support the flexibility of your brain. It is important for the different parts of your brain to be in good communication with each other—in other words, well integrated and working together. The left and right sides of your brain have different functions, biases, and tendencies. For example, the left is more intellectual while the right is more feeling. Optimal functioning occurs when both sides play a role and communicate with each other. If you are too stuck in your right brain, your emotions may override good judgment. If you are too locked into the left side of your brain, your thinking may interfere with your awareness and addressing of feelings. Neuroscientist Dan Siegel says that integration is at the heart of well-being.

NOVELTY, CREATIVITY, AND YOUR BRAIN

There are three main levels to your brain, as discussed previously: the most primitive or reptilian lower part of the brain, the limbic or mammalian brain just above it, and the cortex or primate part at the top of your brain. You want these three areas to be in communication as well, so that you receive information and respond through the appropriate appraisal of all three areas.

Too much of the time we get hijacked by the lower or survival and emotional centers of the brain. This is typically due to fear or habit patterns. When this happens, the cortex, where our decision-making and other higher functions take place, tends to shut down, cutting off access to more reasoned approaches. The result is a less effective response, along with greater tension and activation of your body as you go into fight-or-flight mode.

Optimal health and brain function are enhanced when the two sides of your brain are integrated, as well as when the three levels of your brain are working in harmony. These next exercises are designed to help you gain the flexibility to move through the different levels of your brain. They will challenge your brain to be flexible, to adjust, and to learn in new ways. This encourages new brain pathways as well as simply awakening the brain out of old patterns. Go to step eleven now.

STEP 11 *Looking at flexibility between levels of your brain*

I will give you three different scenarios or visualizations. One will trigger a survival response of the lower center of your brain, one will trigger an emotional response of the middle level of your brain, and one will encourage a more cognitive/creative response of the most evolved level of your brain. For this step on your path, I'd like you to fully imagine being in each of these scenarios and then shuttle between them.

Take about sixty seconds with each visualization and rotate through each one at least two times. Through this shuttling process, your brain will learn to let go and shift gears more readily. As a result, you will have greater flexibility of control when you are out in the real world.

Primitive response visualization:
Imagine walking down a dark and deserted street only to hear footsteps behind you. As you speed up your pace, the steps behind you speed up as well. You walk faster, but the footsteps behind you are getting closer. You break into a run.

Emotional response visualization:
Imagine someone in your life being disrespectful toward you. Perhaps that person is not paying attention, or perhaps he is cheating you. Or it might be something that has actually happened, causing you to be angry. Allow your emotions to flow.

Decision-making visualization:
Imagine getting into your car, about to drive to a distant location. Figure out the route you will need to take (without the help of a GPS).

Now shuttle through these three visualizations. Stay with each long enough for a full experience.

By switching between these three very different experiences involving the three levels of your brain, you are encouraging your brain to shift gears and, by doing so, you become more capable of shifting gears under more difficult circumstances. You are also further encouraging the process of brain flexibility and integration.

FLOW, FEAR, AND RESISTANCE

Flow is an optimal state of being, described by psychologist Mihaly Csikszentmihalyi. (I dare you to pronounce his name.) This state has similar qualities to being on The Path. It's a state of consciousness where one is totally absorbed in what he or she is doing. In other words, you are not distracted by unfinished business, fears, or self-consciousness. It incorporates focus as well as being in harmony with mind and body. When you are in flow you are engaging effortlessly, with the awareness that something special is occurring.

Flow is frequently associated with peak performance, but I prefer a broader concept of optimal functioning that anyone can achieve. In this state, you are feeling fully alive and in tune with what you are doing. You are also fully resilient, as your body utilizes the exact amount of energy that is needed for the behavior—no more and no less. It also puts you on The Path toward success.

Flexibility is a necessary ingredient for the experience of flow. It's about being attuned with the environment such that there is an intimate connection. You are ready and available for instantaneous feedback, and you use that feedback to make the best choice and adjustment. The other day as I was stepping off the sidewalk into the street, my foot landed partly over a hole. My foot and leg began to twist as there was support under only half my foot. In that moment of awareness I relaxed that leg, falling forward and then catching myself with the other foot. This avoided placing too much weight on the unevenly supported foot. Thanks to my presence and flexibility in that moment, I believe I avoided the possibility of spraining my ankle—or worse.

Presence and flexibility are inhibited by fear, defensiveness, and resistance. Fear or simply resistance (such as stubbornness or "I want to do it my way") creates a guard or tension. That, in turn, interferes with your connection with the contact boundary discussed in the last pillar of resilience. In step twelve you have an opportunity to experiment with flow.

STEP 12   *A two-handed experiment of flow*

Let's use your left hand to represent you and your right hand to represent your environment. Hold up your hands facing each other.

Allow your hands to come together—just barely touching. Begin moving your hands in a back-and-forth or up-and-down rhythm in which your hands are in continuous relationship.

Allow your right hand—the environment—to lead, and your left hand, representing you, to be flexible and thus able to closely follow the right hand. Allow yourself to get into a creative flow. Next, add some resistance or tension. In other words, reduce your left hand's flexibility or imagine your left hand becoming stubborn, and notice the change in the experience. You might observe that there is now some jerkiness, stops and starts, and an interruption of the flow that you had at first.

This two-handed experiment of flow can demonstrate what happens in real life when you are not in tune with your environment. For example, you might be walking down the street, as in my example, and trip on an irregularity in the sidewalk. Flow might be the difference between breaking an ankle or having the flexibility and quick mental and physical recovery to help you react and adjust before your ankle breaks. Do step thirteen now.

STEP 13   *Think of a time or situation in your life when you felt like you were in flow.*

It might have been during a physical exercise or sport; it might have been in a business negotiation or while embarked on a creative process. Recall the experience right now, in as great a detail as possible, including your felt sense—the feeling of the experience. Notice how you are totally absorbed in the moment, with no worries.

Acknowledge the benefits and importance of such an experience and how this demonstrates your capability to achieve it under the right circumstances. By doing this—by being flexible and shifting into this state right now—you are increasing your capability to shift into flow at other times.

Sometime during the day today, create a zone of safety, as described previously. This is where you say, "For the moment, I'm completely safe. Nothing bad can happen to me for the next fifteen or twenty minutes, and thus I can completely let go of any fears. I can let down my guard and truly be in the moment." Then use that time to visualize going into the flow state around some preferred activity.

MENTAL FLEXIBILITY

The other day I was standing on a hill overlooking the ocean and there was a chilly breeze. I felt cold and my first thought was that I wasn't wearing enough warm clothes for the conditions. I was far from home and thus couldn't get another jacket. I decided to see what I could do to alter my experience. I imagined that it was a very hot day and that a cool breeze would be refreshing. As I reframed and imagined these conditions, I was able to experience the breeze much differently. I did not feel as cold, and I was able to continue my walk without discomfort.

I realize that if it were too cold, I might not have been able to do this. But within certain limits, I was able to shift my perception of the conditions. Perhaps you have heard of people walking over hot coals in their bare feet after getting into the right mental and emotional state. It demonstrates the power of our minds and the power of mental flexibility. You, too, can engage this ability. Even if you don't realize you have this power, you can develop it simply through practice. Notice where you are right now. Perhaps you are sitting in your bedroom or living room. Perhaps you are in the library or another public place. How are you feeling?

Are you happy? Perhaps you are not feeling so great emotionally. Go to steps fourteen and fifteen now.

STEP 14 *Ability to reframe; mind over matter*

Now I'd like to do an experiment: Imagine that you are in the room of a hotel that is right on the beach in Hawaii. Take a moment to truly imagine that right outside your door there are palm trees, the ocean, and balmy weather, and when you finish reading you are going to walk outside. What does this mental shift do for your mood and anticipation?

STEP 15 *Shift your mindset*

Think of your day or a current problem you are having difficulty with. It might be with another person or with a task. Try changing your mindset to experience the situation differently. For example, imagine fully trusting yourself or imagine that you have total self-confidence. Another approach is to think of someone very successful. For the moment, imagine being that person, getting ready to tackle, or rather, embrace this challenge. Approach this difficulty from one of these perspectives and notice if it makes a difference.

Conversely, imagine that the world is a more accepting, abundant, and loving place. And that this is how you will be received or how your work will be received. Give yourself the opportunity, the psychological space, to fully appreciate and be in this perspective. Notice if this flexing of your mental perspective makes a difference in how you feel. Try using this approach throughout your day today.

This exercise begins to address what I see as a common perspective of a dangerous world filled with judgmental people, where you are more likely to be rejected than accepted. This is a subject addressed in pillar five. Our goal right now is to establish greater flexibility in mental perspective. I will suggest that shifting into a more positive and optimistic perspective is not only healthier, but it also will enhance your performance and flow as you exhibit less resistance or guardedness. For those of you who say, "Wait a minute. Again with this Pollyanna approach that just isn't realistic," hear me out. Continual guardedness and negative expectations don't enhance your security or improve your outcome—just the opposite.

Remember, what is needed during pressure or a dangerous situation is the calm focus described in previous chapters: the one-finger exercise #2. This is the new stress response I have been encouraging you to develop, to actually reengineer your stress response to be more appropriate to your real needs and to a modern world that doesn't reward excessive muscle tension or higher blood pressure. Being flexible with your mental perspective is an important step forward.

One of my clients grew up in a very dysfunctional home. His father left when he was five years old, and he never knew if his mother was going to hit him for the most minor transgression. They lived on the edge of poverty in Philadelphia, and at an early age he learned that he couldn't rely on anyone. He succeeded by being very vigilant, by expecting the worst and preparing for it. When he began seeing me, in his fifties, he was very successful but also very stressed. He had developed high blood pressure and had difficulty sleeping.

My goal with Mike wasn't to change him from someone who was always hypervigilant to someone who was laid back. His approach did have value and had contributed to his success. But he didn't need to be in this mode all the time. He didn't have to be vigilant on weekends or in the evenings. And even during his workday he needed to discriminate moments to be on the alert and those moments when he could let down his guard and release his tension. So the work was about being flexible with his approach: at times being vigilant and calm and at other times letting go, relaxing, and not worrying. The key to this flexibility was being able to discern, to determine when each approach was most appropriate and be able to make the shift. Where can you make this kind of discrimination and go into a more relaxed mode? Do step sixteen now.

STEP 16   *Vigilance flexibility*

For the next twenty-four hours, consciously flex your level of vigilance or guardedness. Find the moments that you can, at least momentarily, let down your guard, soften your gaze, and breathe slowly.

EMOTIONAL FLEXIBILITY

Which emotions do you find yourself most in touch with? Or I might say, which feeling states do you get stuck in? Sadness? Depression? Which do you experience the least? Joy? Excitement? Many situations can cause an upset. It might be a rejection or some type of failure. Here, emotional flexibility is being able—after a certain point—to interrupt and shift out of the negative feelings into a more positive emotional state. Flexibility is also being able to move beyond your current boundaries and allow yourself to experience joy and happiness. Right now I'd like to take you through a process to practice this concept of emotional flexibility. Let's go to step seventeen.

STEP 17   *Practice emotional flexibility to release an upset*

Visualize a recent experience in which you were disappointed, rejected, or that otherwise triggered some form of upset. Perhaps you are still feeling the effects.

We are going to use this experience to practice emotional flexibility and releasing upsets.

Remember this situation by reviewing it, visualizing it in your head. As best you can, allow yourself to drop into the emotional state caused by this experience.

Ask yourself after a few minutes, "Do I want to continue feeling upset?" (This already suggests that you have a choice.) "Have I suffered enough with this negative emotion?"

"What would I prefer feeling? What would be a more positive feeling?"

Identify an image, person, or situation that can give you or remind you of this more positive feeling.

Now, allow yourself to fall into this state of more positive feeling. I know this is only an experiment, but as you have been learning, visualizations and dress rehearsal all contribute to growing new and more positive brain circuits and behaviors. They help you expand your boundaries. These experiences help you make a shift and thus make the process of shifting easier.

FLEXIBILITY IN WHERE YOU PLACE YOUR FOCUS

As I review how my clients get stuck, it frequently stems from the tendency to focus on what might go wrong, the potential negative outcome. Then it's about guarding against this negative outcome occurring. Another way this happens is by clients placing all their focus on the obstacles in the way of achieving their goals. It's like jumping into a pool for a swim. If you focus on how cold the water will feel as you enter, you might never do it. If you focus on how much fun it will be once you are in, then the few seconds of coldness will not stop you.

This dichotomy illustrates something else that's very important. I'm assuming you would like to have more joy, happiness, and excitement in your life. The most common way this happens is by focusing on what can give you joy; in other words, various positive outcomes to your actions. When the obstacle or what might go wrong is attended to, the result is likely to be depression, because there is no room for the experience of joy and excitement. As mentioned previously, you have to focus "above the line" into the positive half of life's experience to make them more likely to occur. Go to step eighteen now.

STEP 18 *Shift focus to let go of negativity*

Identify a situation with which you are currently having some difficulty. Notice the negative thinking—about what can go wrong or the obstacles you face.

For a moment, shift your focus. Concentrate on the positives, on what can go right and what can be achieved. Allow yourself to engage fully in this positive experience.

Use this more positive perspective to motivate you and move past your stuck point.

SHIFTING YOUR BELIEF IN YOURSELF AND YOUR SELF-CONCEPT—FOCUSING ON WHAT'S POSSIBLE

Whether you think that you can or you
think you can't, you're right.
—Henry Ford (1863–1947)

It only takes a small shift for revolutionary changes to take place in your life! And this shift begins with your belief system. At the beginning of chapter one, I discussed grasping the possible. I used running the four-minute mile as an example of the effects of your belief system. After Roger Bannister became the first person to run the mile in under four minutes, ten other runners did it within a year. Before Bannister accomplished this feat, it was thought to be impossible.

I've been talking about your fixed patterns, your primitive Gestalts, and how they limit your growth, placing a ceiling over your head. They do this by predetermining what you think you are capable of and what you are not, and what actions you are willing or not willing to take. As we've discussed, this approach is also referred to as a fixed mindset.

Earlier in this chapter I had you create an imaginary circle and place yourself in the center of this circle. The circle circumscribes the boundary between what is you and what is not you. You then did an exercise to flex your boundary. You may have heard your boundary referred to as an invisible ceiling; but in fact, it's more than just a ceiling that limits. For example, if you believe you don't have confidence or you can't learn a skill, it gets in the way of you becoming confident or learning that skill. These goals will sit outside of the boundary that demarcates what is you and what is not you. I want you to continue developing flexibility in your beliefs. As you know, this is what's referred to as a growth mindset. It says, "I'm capable of learning and growing."

This approach begins by visualizing this boundary that surrounds you as being movable and having the potential to be expanded outward. In other words, your boundary—who you are—is flexible. Do steps nineteen and twenty now.

STEP 19 *Focus on possibilities*

Think of something you want to achieve but you've had difficulty getting beyond a certain point. Or it might be a goal that appears daunting. We might even say you are limited by your image of yourself—who you are and what's not you.

Instead of focusing on not knowing if you can do it, can you say that there is a possibility that you can do it? And if so, can you visualize yourself as a person capable of achieving this? Let's explore this possibility.

Identify all the reasons you can achieve this goal, or think of a positive outcome and all the reasons it's possible for you to achieve it. Next, picture yourself already having achieved the goal. Imagine this in as great a detail as possible, including how you would feel. From this vantage point, look back and see the path you took to get to this goal.

Now focus on the intention of finding a way to make this outcome a reality.

STEP 20   *Making a choice*

When you get ready to take action, remember the result of this exercise. Then be aware that you have a choice. You can focus on the difficulty or why you might not be able to achieve this goal, or you can choose to focus on the fact that it is possible for you to achieve it. I call this a "choice point."

And these points are in front of you every moment. Start noticing the choice points in each day and in your life. Always choose the positive choice: the "it's possible" choice.

Whatever quality you want to consider, its achievement and growth are more likely to occur when you focus on the possibility, when you focus on moving beyond your existing boundary and pushing your boundaries out. You will be better able to engage with the world from this perspective and increase your chances for success. One of the byproducts of this process will be a growth in your self-confidence inside your boundary. This will serve to enhance your trust in yourself, further enhancing the achievement of your goals.

GROWING YOUR CONFIDENCE AND TRUST IN YOURSELF

Much of the time we will either consciously or unconsciously make a statement about ourselves such as: "I have no confidence" or "I don't have any willpower." We say it as if it were black or white: Either I have it or I don't have it—as if it's something that is either there or not there. In other words, we are back to that fixed mindset. Even when we do see shades of gray, we still frame it in a fixed way: This is what I have, this is who I am, or this is who I'm not. The result is a difficulty in seeing the path—or The Path for shifting into a greater sense of yourself. Let's find a different way of holding these qualities such that The Path for growth is visible and possible.

In pillar four we looked at the activation/relaxation gradient, particularly in relationship to sleep. If you are having difficulty falling asleep, it can feel like this huge chasm between being awake and being asleep. If this were reframed in terms of a continuum from the highest levels of activation going down to the deepest levels of calm and relaxation, where sleep can occur, immediately a path materializes. "OK, instead of this big chasm, all I have to do is gradually, step by step, lower my arousal level. If I have patience, I'll eventually get there."

Let's take confidence as an aspect of your self-concept. Let's take it because it plays such a pivotal role in your life and can be used as a good example here as well. No matter what, I'd say that you have some confidence. There are some things you know you can do. There are some situations you know you can handle. At the same time, there are other situations where you don't feel confident. In other words, you can place yourself somewhere on the continuum of confidence. Now, go to steps twenty-one and twenty-two on The Path.

STEP 21 | *Accepting your level of confidence in order to increase it*

Once again imagine the circle that surrounds who you are. At this time we will focus only on your sense of self-confidence. How would you describe your confidence level?

Now I'd like you to say what sits outside your circle with respect to self-confidence. How are you not confident? Where or what don't you feel capable of doing or achieving?

To begin with, it's important to let go of judgments around this issue. So I'd like you to be accepting of this level of confidence. Remember the lessons of the first pillar: Coming from a place of acceptance is the shortest route to success. It also puts you smack-dab in the middle of The Path.

Think about your boundary as being flexible so that it's susceptible to moving out and thus incorporating greater levels of confidence.

STEP 22   *Take the challenge to grow your self-confidence*

Identify some task you can do—perhaps with some difficulty, something that's just at the edge of your boundary that stretches you.

We can call this your challenge. To accept this challenge opens you to growth and increasing self-confidence and self-trust.

Make a commitment to do this in the next few days even though it might be uncomfortable. Plan and schedule a time to do it.

When you follow through with this difficult but doable task, make sure you fully take it in. Make sure you appreciate yourself and recognize that you pushed your boundary of confidence and self-trust out a bit further.

This is how you shift your belief system, your confidence level, and your trust in yourself: taking actions right at the edge of your boundary, accepting the challenge and doing what's difficult but necessary, and then appreciating this effort. And note: Even if the action doesn't result in total success, it's still important to appreciate the effort, the courage it took to take this step.

DANCING WITH THE SOURCE—FINDING YOUR RHYTHM

Non-duality is a perspective that says that everything is one and that all distinctions, all separations, are an illusion. It's like we are all drops of water that, when placed in the ocean, meld into each other. But this is difficult to imagine as we all are aware of the skin that separates us from the world. It's very difficult—if not impossible—for us to imagine this "oneness" that is described in many ancient teachings.

But if you can't quite grasp this universality of existence, it might be possible to imagine that there is an interconnectedness among everything in our universe. For example, right now you are breathing in air; it enters your lungs, where there is an exchange of gases, and then you breathe this air out into the world. Where was this air before it entered your body and where did it go? If you are in a room with other people or even animals, there is a good chance that particles of air that you breathe in were inside another organism moments before. Would you call this interconnectedness? And we have already discussed how your heartbeat can be detected in the brain waves of someone close to you.

What's the advantage of a perspective of non-duality? Well, the first and most obvious is that by imagining this new perspective, you are engaging the process of flexibility as you attempt to make a shift from the dualistic and separateness of all things in life. Another is that a non-duality perspective immediately puts you outside your own boundary circle: If everything is one, then you are what's outside your circle as well as what's inside. Wow, that was easy, wasn't it? Well, maybe it's not so easy.

When I tried this myself, I actually shuttled between these two perspectives—separateness and oneness—as I tried holding them both at once. And I found that I could sense a rhythm I was creating in this process. By staying with it, I was able to feel a sense of wholeness. When this happened, it had a very positive effect on me. Let's try an experiment to get a feeling for this. Go to steps twenty-three through twenty-six.

STEP 23 *Experiencing non-duality*

Take your hand and hold it up in front of you. Observe your hand—your fingers, your knuckles, your wrist, your palm. Now notice everything but your hand. Shuttle back and forth between your hand and everything else. Now try looking at your hand and everything else at the same time.

STEP 24   *Experiencing a rhythm with yourself and the world*

Notice yourself. This may seem like a strange request, but simply be aware of yourself; notice the space inside your skin. Now shift your awareness to what's outside of yourself, of your skin. Shuttle back and forth—within and without. See if you can get into a rhythm as you shift your awareness.

STEP 25   *Being one with the world*

Imagine everything that you notice in this exercise being one: what is outside and what is inside you. Do this by playing with or dancing with the rhythm of shifting back and forth—until the two perspectives appear to meld into one. Don't judge yourself; simply play with this exercise.

STEP 26   *Experiencing flexibility and levels of your boundary*

Let's try doing this another way: Notice yourself, the space within your skin. Next, expand this awareness out slightly to incorporate what might be considered your "aura," a subtle energy field that surrounds you. Some refer to this as your psychological space, or the buffer between you and the rest of the world. Get a sense of this larger you. Next expand still further to everything surrounding you that you are able to see.

In other words, expand your personal boundary to incorporate your surroundings. Let's take this another step and imagine your boundary expanding to larger and larger areas—your community, your country, the entire Earth. Keep moving this boundary out beyond the solar system and the Milky Way galaxy. Keep expanding until your boundary takes in the entire universe. Play with these different levels of boundaries. There isn't a right or wrong; simply experiment with this process. Each step represents progress in your growing ability to be flexible.

I have taken you through many levels of flexibility in this eighth pillar of resilience and success. I've concluded with the experience of a oneness with everything, a big leap in flexibility. Through this process, you have played with and further altered the boundary of your primitive Gestalt. Indeed, you have made that boundary permeable and less and less recognizable from the original at the beginning of the book. As I guide you onto The Path, you are engaging the process of growth, healing, and success. Ultimately, you are establishing a more mature and healthy Gestalt pattern.

SIGNPOST

- You have "stalked your pattern" and identified limiting beliefs or thinking.
- You have also identified positive characteristics within the boundary of who you are.
- You have identified qualities you want that are, for the moment, outside your boundary.
- You have imagined that your boundary is flexible.
- You have experimented with doing routine behaviors with your non-dominant hand.
- You have used visualization to become more comfortable with something you have been anxious about.
- You have used visualizations to become more flexible in shifting between the three levels of your brain.
- You used the two-handed experiment to experience levels of "flow."
- You experimented with reframing, flexibility of perspective, and mindset to gain greater control over your emotional state and foster emotional flexibility.
- You experimented with shifting into a positive thinking pattern and one of possibilities.
- You took steps—took the challenge—to expand your boundaries out into new territory.
- You experimented with your focus to being one with what's outside of yourself.

CHAPTER 15

PILLAR NINE

Power: The Ability to Get Things Done

When most people talk about power, they are referring to wealth, business success, fame, military strength, or political control. But when these come at the expense of health, relationships, or the loss of your soul, it is a hollow victory. The Dalai Lama says that the ultimate purpose of life is to be happy. And it's hard to argue with the statement that the achievement of power is only real power if it's accompanied by happiness and a concern for others; that it's linked to relationships and giving back.

True power takes into account all nine pillars of my model, with this—my ninth pillar—defined as the ability to get things done. In fact, Figure 3 on page 332 presents a reframing of my model into what I refer to as the "pyramid of power," with power sitting on the shoulders of the other eight pillars. The Path has been building a sound and sturdy foundation, or grounding, that incorporates heart and soul.

Now, from this foundation, you are able to thrust out into the world and be successful—while maintaining balance and resilience. I purposely define and teach power in a way that minimizes the possibility of it being abused. In the world today, power is abused too much of the time—usually by taking advantage of, or by using it against, others—although I can make a case that there is also a personal soul-wounding aspect. The more power one has, the greater the potential for it to be abused. Think of a rocket ship taking off, with the huge explosion of energy required to lift it off its platform. The slightest shift off course will be exaggerated by the magnitude of the power.

In pillar three, I introduced the concept of "the source." It's not an original notion about life and the universe but a very ancient notion about the unity of everything. From this perspective, all energy and power originate from this oneness. And the amount of energy that's available is tremendous. Think of the power released by the smashing of infinitesimally small atoms, which gives us atomic energy.

You and I are the instruments through which this energy flows. How your "instrument" is healed, and how open and how deeply you

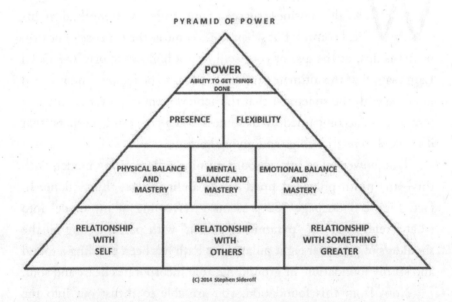

PYRAMID OF POWER

POWER
ABILITY TO GET THINGS DONE

PRESENCE   FLEXIBILITY

PHYSICAL BALANCE AND MASTERY   MENTAL BALANCE AND MASTERY   EMOTIONAL BALANCE AND MASTERY

RELATIONSHIP WITH SELF   RELATIONSHIP WITH OTHERS   RELATIONSHIP WITH SOMETHING GREATER

(C) 2014 Stephen Sideroff

FIGURE 3 | Pyramid of Power: showing how the ninth pillar of resilience and success sits atop of the other eight pillars

can reach inside determine how much energy is available. How it is tuned determines how effectively and how purely you will use it. When power is exerted outside of my model, some of that energy contributes to imbalance, strain, and, ultimately, overwhelm or burnout. Your instrument needs to be developed, maintained, and then played in a specific manner to get the best and most powerful vibrational sound. Early in this book I explained how our evolution and our early training resulted in us being improperly tuned and tuned to the wrong lessons. The more you have been on The Path, you have been optimally tuning your "instrument." As you have progressed through my program, the more you are now able to experience and employ your power to mutually benefit you and others.

POWER AND RESILIENCE

On the most basic of levels, resilience is about the ongoing assessment and restoration of personal balance in all areas—physical, emotional, mental, and spiritual—while learning new lessons. Where there isn't balance, resilience is the ability to notice the lack of balance—and the intention, ability, and follow-through to restore balance. The greater your resources and capacity for following through, the more easily you are able to restore balance. In addition, as your sense of your capability and self-confidence increases—by setting intentions, following through, reaching goals, and achieving success—your concerns and worry about life challenges will decrease. This is when you feel in control of your life and life challenges. This is truly being on The Path, and this is what I mean by "power."

Power implies mastery in life. It signifies a willingness—indeed, a desire—to do what is necessary to achieve your goals, to take an active and responsible role in your life. And it results in the growth of confidence and self-trust. This reduces stress. As we have come to the ninth pillar of resilience and success, we are also at the pillar that most addresses success.

GROWING POWER

It's important at the start to realize that the ability to get things done—power—is not an all-or-nothing ability; it also is not static or fixed. It's important that you don't lock yourself in by saying, "I don't have any power" or even "I don't have much power." As with other abilities we have worked with, there is a continuum here. As you have gone through the resilience and healing process of the prior fourteen chapters, you have already made important changes to your self-image and beliefs about yourself that have enhanced your power. But you still might not be objective when it comes to recognizing your power capacity. It's usually much greater than you think. We want to do as objective an appraisal of abilities as possible but then also to be accepting of wherever you are. Our goal here is to be OK with where you are currently—your foundation (and not feel like you are lacking and have to dig yourself out of a hole, which creates greater strain)—with the intention of growing your power. This will result in greater trust in yourself, more confidence, and increased personal capacity.

In addition, it's also important to recognize that our society and our families do a poor job of helping us transition from children to adults capable of holding power. More specifically, there wasn't a conscious process to help you make this leap. You struggle, you cope, you try to do it—usually on your own, as your parents are also struggling with this issue. Indigenous cultures recognize that help is needed in this process. These societies have developed rituals around the process of "transfer of power." Through this process, the adolescent learns the ways of power and gets permission to own his or her power. This, in fact, is demanded of the individual. These rituals help turn over power from one generation to the next.

My experience with most people I've worked with in Western culture is that the parents themselves don't feel powerful. They either hold on to power jealously, or unconsciously, they give their offspring the message not to challenge them, not to "get too big for your britches," as the father of one of my clients told him.

As a result of these messages and this missing process, you reach adulthood without feeling powerful. You feel too young to take on this mantle of maturity. You try valiantly, but since your primitive Gestalt says you can't, you then feel like an impostor when you are successful. For many, this says, "I'm not powerful; I must not be OK." And this perpetuates the sense of being young. Many car manufacturers thrive on this inadequacy as we buy bigger or more expensive cars to compensate. Do steps one through three on The Path now.

STEP 1 *Accepting empowering messages from childhood*

Review your childhood relationship with your parents, particularly your father. Can you identify messages from them, either verbally or through their actions, that were empowering? Perhaps they encouraged you to engage in a hobby, sport, or go further in school. Perhaps they showed approval of your efforts. Take a moment to acknowledge these positive messages.

STEP 2 *Identifying undermining childhood messages*

Can you identify messages that were discouraging: limiting, negative judgments, or critical statements, such as "You'll never get it," "Why can't you do it right?" or "You're not very smart." Perhaps it was lack of any approval—the silence speaking loudly. Or perhaps they compared you to the child next door: "Why can't you be like so and so?"

STEP 3 *Being your own healthy parent*

What if you were to imagine being your own good parent? If you truly wanted your son or daughter—meaning you—to be successful, to be empowered and supported, what would you say that's a true reflection of your abilities? How can you speak to yourself in an encouraging way? Speak that way to yourself right now.

RENEWING YOUR INTENTIONS AND MOTIVATIONS

Let's reconnect with your motivations and intentions for resilience and success, and now, more specifically, for feeling powerful, for owning your power, for growing your ability to get things done. You might want to review some of the notes you took at the beginning of this program when intention and commitment were first discussed. Perhaps some of your motivations have changed as a result of this program.

What's important to you? Where do you want to get to? What do you want to achieve? And what is your cutting edge, the place on the outskirts of your existing boundary that you need to step beyond for your success? The clearer you are with these intentions, the easier it is to be on The Path. We have been looking at these issues with respect to you and your relationships. We now also want to include your motivations with career, purpose, or goals. But don't get stuck because you can't identify some grand purpose. Getting things done can involve something as simple as being able to complete your taxes or build a bookcase. The goal here is to grow your ability to get things done. Whatever you choose to focus on is simply an exercise in examining and enhancing your process. You can begin anywhere. Do steps four through nine now.

STEP 4   *Identify something you want to achieve*

Identify something you want to achieve. It can be tomorrow, this year, or it can have a longer horizon. This can be a new goal or one you have been struggling with for a long time.

STEP 5   *What is your motivation?*

Why is this important to you? Is it for financial security, personal satisfaction, helping others, some other purpose, or all of the above? Take a few minutes to sit with this motivation and allow it to be fully accepted within you.

STEP 6 *Find your passion*

How strong is your intention around this goal? How important is it and how hard are you willing to work to achieve it? How much are you willing to overcome in order to achieve this end? The more you can bring up your passion and your desire, the more you will be able to overcome your primitive Gestalt patterns of fear and self-judgment, and be successful.

STEP 7 *Commit to taking action*

Make a commitment to follow through and take action, to do whatever it takes to achieve success with this goal. Write this action into your schedule or appointment book. Remember, there still might be some fear present. The goal is to reach inside and find enough courage to overcome the fear.

STEP 8 *Do a dress rehearsal*

Take a moment and visualize your action and your goal already being achieved. Let yourself accept the result in as great a detail as possible. Give those brain circuits of success a head start with this dress rehearsal.

STEP 9 *Create an affirmation to ensure success*

Create an affirmation that states you have already achieved this goal. Add this to the other affirmations that you read in the morning, throughout the day, and before you go to sleep.

The purpose of imagining already having achieved success is to activate and accentuate your motivation for this task. The more motivated you are, the greater the likelihood you will tackle obstacles and break through old boundaries to achieve success. Once you tap in to this motivation, you continue the process of ensuring success by identifying your intention and commitment. Intention takes your motivation and gives it a specific direction. It also mobilizes unseen forces in your world in support of your goals. This is facilitated by your commitment, or your promise, that you will follow through and not drop the ball. Remember what Johann Wolfgang von Goethe said, "When you commit to action with boldness, the universe conspires to support you." Be bold and call on the universe to support you.

Some people have great difficulty at this point. If you set too big or difficult a goal, fear of failure may interrupt the process. If you don't know all of the steps necessary to achieve your goal, your uncertainty can lead to procrastination or giving up. So make sure you have established a reasonable yet challenging goal. If it's too overwhelming, break it into smaller and more doable goals. If you are unsure of the path, of all the steps in the process to reach your goal, you either need more information or the support of a mentor, teacher, or some other help. Again, don't let this stop the process. It just means your path will include information gathering and/or the help of others. Do steps ten, eleven, and twelve now.

STEP 10 *Feel into your achievement*

Make a verbal statement right now that helps you own your motivation for achieving your goal. This statement might look like: "This is a great achievement; I'm really going to go for it" or "When I imagine reaching this goal, it feels so good that I must do whatever it takes to accomplish it."

STEP 11 *Establishing and maintaining an intention*

I'd like you to prepare to state your intention to reach this goal. This preparation involves all parts of yourself being in alignment that this goal is important and that you want to achieve it. Make sure you can say that you deserve to achieve it. Then feel it in your heart and body and know it in your mind. The preparation includes sending out a message to the universe that you are setting this intention and not hiding from it.

Once having done this, state your intention out loud. Also, write it down.

STEP 12 *Establishing and maintaining your commitment*

As noted above, your commitment is your promise to do whatever it takes to achieve this goal. This means you must be willing to take actions that might be difficult, uncomfortable, and perhaps even scary in order to achieve the goal.

Make a statement about your commitment and promise right now. Schedule your next action steps toward reaching your goal.

RECONNECTING WITH YOUR FOUNDATION

No matter where you begin in this process of growing your power, you have a foundation, a place from which to anchor yourself. Whatever this foundation is, it needs to be appreciated so you get the greatest benefit for taking your next step. How you get stuck, as mentioned previously, is when you focus on what you aren't or what you don't have rather than what is.

One of my clients who had a particularly difficult childhood was hard-pressed to identify successes in her life. It just felt like she barely survived, without any recognition from her parents. Very little that she did seemed to make them happy. So much of the time they were yelling at each other or at her and her siblings. In our work together, what she discovered was that simply making it through her very difficult childhood of huge stresses, without good support from her parents, was in itself a major accomplishment and demonstrated great ingenuity.

As we delved further into her experience, she began to identify important abilities that served her. She had become very good at reading the expressions on her parents' faces to know what to expect, to know if she should quickly get out of the house and away from a potential emotional storm. She became good at negotiating. She had discovered ways of appeasing her parents. Up to that point, she had seen all these "abilities" as being sneaky, as "getting away with things." As an adult they contributed to her feeling like she was not OK and was simply pulling the wool over people's eyes. But in fact, she was placed into a very difficult and unsupportive environment. On her own, she figured out how to navigate choppy waters and stormy seas to get through to adulthood. Now, with this new perspective, she began to appreciate and accept her gifts and abilities.

What are the planks in the flooring of your foundation? What can you stand on in terms of your abilities? And what do your successes demonstrate in terms of skills and gifts? Go to steps thirteen through seventeen on The Path now.

STEP 13   *Reflecting on your history*

What are some of your successes that you previously dismissed by saying that you were lucky, that anyone could have done it, or by using some other way of deflecting the positive?

Be creative and thus very inclusive with all examples of your positive results.

Keep going—don't stop. Search a little deeper to find more of your abilities, gifts, and successes.

STEP 14   *Accept your achievements*

Take a moment simply to breathe and, as you breathe in, take in and accept these achievements. Own them.

STEP 15   *Identify one or more of your successes*

I want to help you identify that part of yourself that is the source of your successes and your strength. For some of you this might be a very big part, and for others it may be small and hard to find inside yourself. You will recall engaging in a similar process within the first pillar.

Take the successes you have just identified. The specifics are not as important as simply being able to remember a time or place where you followed through and achieved success. Don't get hung up by minimizing the experience. Any level of achievement is sufficient for our purposes. As you learned in pillar five, it's about focusing on the positive and allowing yourself to feel good about the successful aspects of your behavior.

STEP 16 *Identify your abilities that led to these successes*

Take a moment to appreciate everything that you did to make this a success. This includes your decision-making, your persistence and hard work, your courage, and your focus. Again, remember this process is about growing your power. Thus, it's important to accept and appreciate whatever level you are starting at. Allow yourself to feel a sense of competence based on this analysis. This is part of your grounding.

STEP 17 *Internal dialogue*

As we did previously, I'd like you to have a dialogue between the part of you that owns and appreciates these successes and the other part that might be doubting and undermining. The part saying "but" is more likely to dismiss your successes while pointing out your shortcomings. Switch chairs as you change voices. See if you can have the supportive voice be more assertive. Don't give in to the negative voice. Even though it's been with you all your life, you are finally taking a stand and deciding you don't have to listen to it anymore. It is outdated. Ground yourself in the new and healthy voice.

OWNING YOUR POWER

When you can reflect on your history and demonstrate to yourself that you can follow through, that there were times when you didn't let obstacles or fear get in your way, you are demonstrating trust in yourself. Think about how this affects stress. Common amid the stress of anxiety and worry is the fear that you won't be able to take care of business, to handle problems, or to deal with the challenges of life. For the moment, own the power you have demonstrated in the past and in this exercise. Again, don't minimize it; simply appreciate it. Don't say what it isn't. Say what it is. Own your power at whatever level! This will help it grow.

CONFIDENCE AND TRUST IN YOURSELF: CHALLENGE, FOLLOWING THROUGH, AND A POSITIVE ATTITUDE

"Do. Or do not. There is no try," declared Yoda in *The Empire Strikes Back*. There are many good excuses! Sometimes we look to blame someone else for our lack of success. But while excuses give you temporary comfort, they don't get you anywhere. None of them enhance your power. Excuses help you to be comfortable within your existing boundaries. That's OK, but you need to be clear: This won't help you grow or become more powerful. And excuses undermine your confidence and, thus, your resilience.

Much of the time we get stopped not by something we are unable to do but by something that is difficult or uncomfortable—or simply by something we have placed outside of our psychological boundary, as described in the previous pillar. We get stopped by the fear and avoidance of making a mistake, looking silly, or feeling awkward. Yet, these are all ingredients of growth and success! Growth doesn't happen when we do something that's easy or that we did previously. It occurs when we take on the challenge and do what's difficult. Get used to discomfort, because it usually accompanies growth. We call it growing pains.

In their book *Flow in Sports*, Susan Jackson and Mihaly Csikszentmihalyi tell us that growth occurs only when we take on a challenge that includes a level of uncertainty. In other words, when something is easy, with no possibility of failure, there is less of a challenge and, thus, no opportunity for growth.

Each time you take a step toward achievement of a goal, each time you say you are going to do something difficult for you and then follow through, you are enhancing your self-confidence and trust in yourself.

You are telling yourself, "I can count on myself to follow through." This is how you truly grow your self-efficacy. Johann Wolfgang von Goethe said, "Magic is believing in yourself; if you can do that, you can make anything happen."

When you take an *active* role in your life, when you accept challenges, follow through, and then frame the results positively, you are growing your power; you are literally nurturing your confidence. When you shy away from challenges, when you allow fear to govern your behavior, you are reinforcing habit patterns that result in less self-trust and that reduce your power. In fact, you are telling yourself, "I can't trust you to keep your word or to follow through." In other words, you are always either growing power or reinforcing your lack of power. Go now to steps eighteen, nineteen, and twenty on The Path.

STEP 18 *Making a commitment*

Right now make a commitment to take some action you have been putting off. Schedule it on your calendar. Demonstrate to yourself that you can begin to count on yourself.

STEP 19 *Is there an obstacle?*

If you are unable to do this, don't leave it at that! First, identify what's getting in your way. Is it too big a step? Is it too scary? Are you afraid you don't have the necessary skills or knowledge?

STEP 20 *Finding a way to move forward*

Here is where you must make a choice of how to move forward.

1. If it's too big, can you take a smaller step in the process?
2. If it's too scary, can you either get support or go through a visualization—a dress rehearsal—of taking the step in order to make it less scary?

3. If you have identified skills you need but don't have, can you acquire them or find someone with the skills to help you?

4. If you need additional information, can you seek out that information?

5. If none of the above get you closer to taking the step, how can you change your goals and expectations (flexibility) in order to find steps you can take?

Following through in the face of uncertainty and risk is an important concept in my work with elite athletes. Defeat is always a part of the game. One tennis player I worked with got to the point where he wanted to quit. He said to me, "Every time I lose, it shakes my confidence." His focus on the possibility of loss or even mistakes caused him to be hesitant and tense. He wasn't able to play his best, and he wasn't able to improve.

I shared with him a story that took place when I was twenty and a water skiing instructor at a camp on Lake George in upstate New York. Some of the children would get up on two skis and never fall into the water. And then there were those who, almost every time they skied, would fall. But it was these kids who, as the summer progressed, were getting better and better. It was these children who were getting up on one ski and winning all the contests as they got lower and lower to the water when they turned, shooting water sprays higher and higher into the air.

That was when I learned a very important lesson. The children who were pushing themselves to their limits, to the edges of their comfort zone, were the ones learning and getting better. At that point of uncertainty and challenge, growth was occurring. But it was also at those moments that they might and did fall. That was another important lesson the kids learned: Falling wasn't so terrible. And the more they fell, the more it became a routine part of getting better and becoming less fearful. Thomas Edison, the famous inventor, once said, "I have not failed. I've just found ten thousand ways that won't work."

The goal here is to feel powerful. To feel like "I can." Remember, you are rarely assured of getting something right the first time. You will not always do it without errors. The positive attitude of "I can" always takes into account that it might require a number of tries, but "I will do it." With this attitude, you approach new situations with less tension, less fear, and with greater ease. Thus, when you try and don't make it, when you try and it doesn't work out, that's when you need to come from the place of "OK, how do I learn from this effort, to have a better chance the next time" instead of deciding "This is too difficult for me." Remember, resilience is about bouncing forward and learning from each challenge. As Thomas Jefferson once said, "I find that the harder I work, the more luck I seem to have."

RESISTANCE TO POWER: PROCRASTINATION; FEAR OF MISTAKES, EXPOSURE, BEING AWKWARD; AND OTHER WAYS YOU HOLD YOURSELF BACK

Procrastination often occurs because you focus on what can go wrong, the difficulties, or simply the discomforts that are in the way of achievement. A friend of mine loves snow skiing but never goes skiing. He never gives himself the opportunity to experience the joy he feels when he skis. When I ask him why, he recounts all the effort it takes to get the equipment and then get to the mountains. His focus on the obstacles interferes with his motivation and his ability to connect with the pleasures of skiing. So he stays home.

Henry Ford said, "Obstacles are those frightful things you see when you take your eyes off your goal."

Let's return to our two internal voices: the spokesperson for your primitive Gestalt pattern and the newer, more mature, positive voice of wisdom we have been developing. Much of your resistance to growth, to your ability to get things done, resides in the messages from the old voice. Consider some of the possible negative messages: "It's not OK to make a mistake"; "Don't put yourself out there, you will be too

vulnerable"; "It's too uncomfortable or dangerous." Or the more unconscious messages such as, "You don't deserve" or "If you move past your
mother or father, you will be disloyal." Let's go to steps twenty-one and
twenty-two on The Path to address your resistance.

STEP 21   *Gestalt dialogue*

Engage in a dialogue between your two internal voices: the old voice
and the new, more positive, supportive, and loving voice. Allow the
new voice of wisdom to respond to the restrictive messages of danger, exposure, and rejection. Notice in this process that the newer and
healthier voice might begin by trying to defend itself and its position.
When you do this, it's the old voice that is still running the show.

STEP 22   *Nurturing an assertive new and healthy voice*

At some point in the dialogue it's important for the new voice to take
charge and change the paradigm. Instead of defending itself, this new
voice would be more assertive and sound something like this:

"You are holding me back. Your messages are old and outmoded.
They are no longer relevant. It's OK if I make a mistake. I can't keep
worrying about what others will think."

Take a moment now to continue with your dialogue and be more
assertive from the perspective of the new voice of wisdom.

TRANSFER OF POWER: HELPING YOU BREAK THROUGH YOUR CEILING AND OUTMODED LEARNED LESSONS AND LOYALTIES

As I mentioned earlier in this chapter, indigenous cultures have rituals
and procedures to help you transition from a child and adolescent into
an adult prepared to face the world. In contrast, our culture leaves this
to chance. And most of the time our culture holds us back rather than

facilitating the process. I want to address this deficiency right now and help you in the process of taking on the mantle of adulthood, of moving into your power. Follow steps twenty-three and twenty-four of The Path.

STEP 23   *Establishing a ritual to own your power*

I want to guide you through a ritual process to support your full transition into owning your power.

Begin with the one-finger pulse exercise #1: pointer finger on your pulse and going into your deep, calm, rhythmic breathing at six breaths per minute. Bring your awareness into your body and allow yourself to feel at home. Take a moment to appreciate yourself for all that you have done to bring yourself to this point on The Path. Next, and when you can be fully present, go to the end of the chapter and read an excerpt from "The Invitation."

As you read it, experience yourself taking on and owning the messages in each of the phrases. Take these words on as your guide to a complete transition into adulthood and power on The Path.

STEP 24   *Creating your own ritual*

To take this process one step deeper, it would be advantageous for you to create your own ritual of owning your power and fully taking on the role of a powerful adult. You can do this by identifying a time and establishing a safe space. Make it a fully multidimensional experience by identifying some special music to listen to. Create your own personal script that you either read or record and play back during your personal ritual.

ONE MORE FEAR

As I have mentioned, we all have access to tremendous power, the energy that's at the source. The more you open to this possibility—by freeing yourself from your emotional unfinished business and other sources of negativity—the less resistance this energy has to fill and nourish you. But as you open to this energy, there is one more hurdle to its full expression, and that's the discomfort attached to being powerful itself. Here's what Marianne Williamson, author and activist, has to say, which Nelson Mandela quoted:

> Our deepest fear is not that we are inadequate. Our deepest fear is that we are powerful beyond measure. It is our light, not our darkness that most frightens us.

In my own experience of coming into my power, which was accompanied by sensing—on a new level—the full beauty that was all around me, I encountered a new and unfamiliar feeling. My first reaction was to shrink from it, as it had the potential to be overwhelming. I realized that this initial reaction was the unconscious feeling of "Can I hold all this light? Will I burst from it?" And at the time, I did wonder whether I really deserved all this bliss. And here is where I believe a strong foundation, the foundation that we have been working so long at achieving throughout The Path, becomes important. It has prepared you for your gifts to fully blossom and for you to move into your power. Do step twenty-five now.

STEP 25   *Affirming your readiness to own your power*

Create an affirmation that acknowledges your readiness to own your power. Here is an example:

"I am stepping in to my power. I deserve it and I have developed a strong foundation to support this power."

THE PURSUIT OF POWER, ACHIEVING YOUR GOALS, SATISFACTION, AND HAPPINESS

The achievement of goals—getting things done—is a major contributor to personal growth and your success. This, in turn, establishes greater resilience as it increases your capacity to engage with your environment to get results. This increased capacity and confidence results in fewer life situations feeling dangerous or even uncertain. And thus, fewer situations will trigger your stress response.

Pillar nine has required a process that, to some degree, reflects aspects of each of the steps encountered on The Path. This includes establishment of an intention and commitment to a goal, determining a path toward the goal, being supportive of yourself, overcoming fears and taking action, being present and flexible, being persistent, and using feedback to reach your goals. If the goal was thwarted in any way, it then required flexibility and persistence to come up with new approaches until the goal was achieved. This process can refer to the simplest of goals, such as satisfying one's hunger for food, and as complicated as achieving career goals.

Many qualities go into enhancing this component of resilience: awareness of a need, focus, follow-through, persistence, courage, and commitment. Developing your power is about being motivated to push through your fears and being able to manage emotional discomfort in order to get things done. In order to experience life satisfaction.

In this chapter, as with the previous chapter, you have demonstrated your power. Congratulations. The last three chapters are designed to enhance and go deeper with what you have already received. Do step twenty-six now.

STEP 26   *Finding a way to remember being on The Path*

Make sure you establish a method for remembering the importance of every day and following through with every step. They all count! Each becomes a brick in the structure that is your life on The Path.

AN EXCERPT FROM THE INVITATION BY ORIAH, FROM HER BOOK, *THE INVITATION*

It doesn't interest me what you do for a living.
I want to know what you ache for
and if you dare to dream
of meeting your heart's longing.

It doesn't interest me how old you are.
I want to know if you will risk
looking like a fool for love
for your dream
for the adventure of being alive.

I want to know
if you have touched
the centre of your own sorrow
if you have been opened
by life's betrayals
or have become shriveled and closed
from fear of further pain.

I want to know
if you can sit with pain
mine or your own
without moving to hide it
or fade it
or fix it.

I want to know
if you can be with joy
mine or your own
if you can dance with wildness
and let the ecstasy fill you
to the tips of your fingers and toes

without cautioning us
to be careful

I want to know
if you can live with failure
yours and mine
and still stand at the edge of the lake
and shout to the silver of the full moon,
"Yes."

I want to know
if you can be alone
with yourself
and if you truly like
the company you keep
in the empty moments.

SIGNPOST

- You have explored your childhood and identified something that supported your development of power as well as something that interfered with that growth.
- You recognized that power is something that can be developed and increased in yourself.

- You have gone through a process to identify some of your gifts, achievements, and abilities.
- You have taken some time to breathe and take in these messages.
- You have identified a goal, why it's important for you, and your intention and commitment to achieve it.
- You have visualized your goal already being achieved.
- You created a statement reflecting your motivation to achieve your goal.
- You have expressed your intention out loud.
- You have followed through with challenging actions in the service of reaching your goal.
- You have worked through stumbling blocks where they have occurred.
- You have engaged in a dialogue between your old voice and your new voice of wisdom.
- You have become more assertive with your voice of wisdom.
- You have begun reading "The Invitation" and meditating on each phrase.
- You have created your own "coming of age" ritual.
- You have created an affirmation acknowledging your readiness to accept your power.
- You are making every day in your life a masterpiece!

CHAPTER 16

RESILIENT AGING

Longevity and Increasing Your "Healthspan"

I began The Path by exploring and activating your motivations for learning to live with greater resilience. In this chapter I present one additional motivator for your passionate desire to be on The Path. That is: the greater your resilience, the more slowly your body will age. This means you'll live longer before experiencing the deteriorating effects of aging. This is referred to as your healthspan. It could also mean the lessening of physical symptoms you already have been struggling with. In fact, if you have been taking the steps all along The Path, you probably have already recognized its benefits in improved health and fewer symptoms.

I'm the same age as Kareem Abdul-Jabbar, a star basketball player for the Los Angeles Lakers during the '70s and '80s. He was part of the team's "Showtime" era, along with Earvin "Magic" Johnson Jr. As long as he was playing professional ball, I felt I was still young. I would say, "Someone my age is playing sports at the highest level." And this would say to me that I was still at the age where peak performance was possible. I specifically chose Kareem, not only because he was great and I was a Lakers fan living in Los Angeles, but also because he was the oldest player in the league when he retired at the age of forty-two.

After Kareem retired, I could no longer use that same story—other than by referring to golfers. Thus, I changed my definition of optimal—and even peak—performance to what it has become today: to live and enjoy life with the greatest functionality and least disability, discomfort, or pain. Resilient or optimal aging signifies the most graceful aging, with minimal organic and functional impairment. It incorporates maximum regeneration while being tuned in to the flow and rhythm of life.

This highlights the ultimate goal of developing resilience, the defining characteristic of what living resiliently means: slowing down the aging process and staying fully functional with fewer symptoms of aging longer into your old age. I can say this in another way: resilience is the optimal and continual regeneration of your body and extending the length of your health, your healthspan.

I have already mentioned that Hans Selye, whose research introduced the concept of human stress, said that aging is simply the sum total of all the stresses we place on our bodies. Let me describe the scientific evidence indicating that this is really true. The focus of this research is on telomeres.

Telomeres occupy the ends of chromosomes. Since DNA at the end of the chromosomes is incapable of replication (during cell division), this information would get lost. Instead, telomeres that cap the ends get lost instead—preserving the DNA. Over time however, with continued shortening of telomeres, the cells age until they can no longer replicate.

The most recent research on cell deterioration has demonstrated that stress speeds up this process. More specifically, psychological distress has been shown to accelerate cellular aging, as indicated by shortened telomere length and reduced telomerase activity. Telomerase is an enzyme that has been shown to repair the telomeres.

A study examining mothers who were caring for chronically ill children found that chronic stress appeared to hasten the shriveling of these telomeres, shortening their life span and speeding the body's deterioration. Dr. Elissa Epel, a University of California, San Francisco, researcher who helped conduct the study, said, "This is the first time that psychological stress has been linked to a cellular indicator of aging in healthy people." And we all have glaring evidence of this fact whenever we compare pictures of our last few presidents from before they took office to after they have been in office a few years. It's hard not to notice the speeding up of the aging process.

The good news is that new research appears to demonstrate that premature aging, as represented by this shortening of the telomeres, can be reversed. Studies are now showing that some of the very exercises you have learned in this book, such as mindfulness and relaxation approaches, increase the telomerase enzyme, which helps to repair the telomeres. This chapter's first step is based on this research, which demonstrates an increase in telomerase with certain visualization exercises. Go to step one now.

STEP 1   *Visualizing the repair of your cells for longer life*

Right now, take a five-minute break to do the following: Get into a comfortable position, turn off your phone, and create a five-minute zone of safety. Using one-finger exercise #1, breathe at six breaths per minute: four seconds in and six seconds out, feeling your pulse and feeling yourself letting go with each exhale. Give yourself a minute of this calming breath, going into greater coherence, and then visualize the nerve cells in your brain.

These cells have fibers, referred to as "dendrites," that receive information from other nerve cells, plus one long fiber, called an "axon," that sends signals out to other cells. The chromosomes can be found in the nucleus of the cell.

Picture telomeres at the endings of the chromosomes (where the fraying occurs), and imagine them bathed in growing amounts of the rejuvenating telomerase enzyme.

Find a rhythm with your breath, almost like waves on the shore: breathe in and visualize the enzyme, breathe out and have it wash over your brain cell nuclei. Imagine that this enzyme is repairing your telomeres, as it bathes your nerve cells.

The shortening of our telomeres is one of what are now referred to as the twelve hallmarks of aging. These are twelve biological processes that contribute to the aging of our cells and our bodies. Chronic stress can be considered the "master hallmark of aging," as it can be shown to impact all twelve. Therefore, as you have been developing greater resilience through the lessons of this book and how to be on The Path, you are helping to slow the aging process.

In pillar three, I discussed the importance of purpose: that the engagement of purpose in your life can potentially rewrite your genetic code. Through the process of evolution and genetic selection, it is likely that our genetic programming limits our lives. Once we pass the age of species usefulness—childbearing and rearing—we are programmed to deteriorate and die, so we no longer use up precious resources and thus further the survival of the species.

I have also discussed how the expression of our genes, referred to as epigenetics, is influenced by the environment—both external and internal. When you develop purpose in your life, you have the potential to influence this expression and send a message to your genetic code through this process of epigenetics: "The species still needs me. I'm doing something that can make a difference." Now, this might not be true if your only purpose is to make money and then consume even more resources. But if you are engaged in a purposeful life, where you are giving back (giving service), this can result in the shifting of the programming and timing of each cell in your body. Go to step two on The Path now.

STEP 2 *Reconfirming purpose*

We know that your thinking and attitude affect your body. Through the science of epigenetics, we are learning that this process will even determine the expression of your genes—how your genetic material develops the cells of your body. By reconfirming your purpose in life on a daily basis, you keep reminding your material body that there is reason for it to sustain itself.

Right now, remember your purpose; take a moment to fully review and express why you awaken in the morning, beyond your daily chores.

Remind yourself of your important reasons for living. It may be improving the lives of others or contributing to restoring the environment.

Put this into another affirmation that you review on a daily basis.

Some of you may have been experiencing the aches and pains that are signs you are not immortal. These symptoms may have been your motivation for wanting to be on The Path. Your symptoms are the effects of what I refer to as "autonomic dysregulation syndrome." This is where your nervous system is out of balance, as I have been discussing. The consequence is a breakdown somewhere in your body. Remember, there is no substitute for practicing some form of relaxation exercise to restore optimal self-regulation. Go to step three on The Path now.

STEP 3 *Practicing self-regulation*

Take ten minutes today—and every day—to do your relaxation-visualization-meditation exercise.

It is my hope that you are sufficiently motivated to keep asking yourself that one question, "Am I on The Path or off The Path?" Continue to follow the guidelines for each of the 9 Pillars of Resilience and Success, and keep working to optimize the process of neurogenesis. This is the key to resilient aging.

SIGNPOST

- You have engaged in a visualization process to heal and repair the cells of your body.
- You have reconfirmed your purpose and noted its importance in a long and healthy life.
- You continue to do a relaxation-visualization-meditation exercise every day.

CHAPTER 17

THE DEEPENING PROCESS

I n this chapter I focus on the ongoing process of letting go and how it can continue opening you to deeper and deeper levels inside yourself. As you face and then eliminate psychological holding, this removes places in your psyche that you have been avoiding and thus have been interfering with your awareness. This furthers the process of awakening. We can compare this process to deepening and strengthening your foundation. As a side benefit, this will allow you to thrust further out into the world for greater success, just as a structure can thrust further up into the sky with a deeper foundation based on strength, solidity, and stability. But more than simply strengthening your foundation, this process will bring deeper meaning and love into your life.

Let's use the broadest meaning of the term "holding on"—the opposite of letting go. Physically, you can hold with a muscle. When you do that, you are tensing, or contracting, the muscle. Think of when you are getting ready to either fight the threat or run from the threat. You tighten muscles in readiness for some explosion. Mentally, you can hold on to an idea, a rule, or a fantasy that no longer serves you or anyone else. Emotionally, you can hold on to your feelings, you can hold on to a loss, you can hold on to a grudge. All these examples, in fact, hold you back. What are you still holding on to? What loss, what muscles, what mistakes, and what resentments? Go to step one on The Path now.

STEP 1 *Identifying what you are still holding on to*

It is important to remember that holding on doesn't hurt the other person or change a past event. It only hurts you. It is a waste of your valuable energy.

Can you decide that it's time for you to let go, so you can channel this energy into more productive efforts to contribute to your success in life? Give yourself this opportunity right now.

The more you let go, the more you can open to the deepest parts of yourself. The results of this opening are a sense of unity, a feeling of bliss, and a feeling of peace. Thus, there is a growing awareness of your interconnectedness (as opposed to feelings of isolation) with those around you and with the world. You may have experienced feelings of bliss when something in life touched you deeply, such that it brought tears to your eyes.

A feeling of peace is the positive summation of all your emotional experience. An analogy is when light shines through a prism: it creates a rainbow of colors. But if you trace this rainbow back to its source, you see white light. If there were a rainbow of all feelings, then peace would be the integration of all of them in the most positive experience of total feeling. It is this full experience that might be compared to unity awareness—an awareness of the interconnectedness of everything. The more you let go, the more you will approach this.

The result of following through with the lessons of The Path is a growing connection with the deepest parts of yourself, along with a deeper connection with those around you and a growing awareness of your interconnection with everything.

Most of us live by the evolutionary process of survival of the fittest. When you come from this perspective, you wind up feeling isolated and separate. A side benefit of shifting onto The Path is a shift from survival of the fittest to living by the Golden Rule, a shift from your animal nature to your spiritual birthright. While survival of the fittest divides and isolates us, the Golden Rule, in its truest sense, pulls us together and fosters a spiritual belief in the interconnectedness of everything and everyone.

To achieve this feeling of peace and the deepening of your sense of self, we will engage in a meditation focused on your heart. As we learned in pillar six, your heart plays a very important role in your experience of feelings. In addition, it plays an important role in the deepening of your consciousness. Puran Bair, meditation teacher and author of *Living from the Heart*, says, "Each person can find the All by going deeply into the Self." And this path goes through the heart. Here is more of what Bair says: "Therefore, to overcome the feeling of separation from 'that world' that people commonly have in 'this world,' you need to experience your heart. Also, to experience your common humanity with people who seem outwardly very different from you, you need the experience of your heart.

"The heart can perform this function of uniting the worlds because it is itself in both worlds: The heart is both physical and spiritual. It regulates your body and directs your mind, and it also represents the core of your Self." Bair also notes, "While Love is abundant in the Source, being the very fabric of the universe, very few can access it there; love is much more easily found in the heart of a human being." Focusing on your heart will help you let go and thus open to the deepest parts of yourself. That expression "follow your heart" has a very deep meaning. Go to step two now.

STEP 2 *Heart meditation*

You might want to memorize this meditation so you can recall it with your eyes closed. Begin with the pointer finger of your right hand on the pulse of your left wrist, as in one-finger relaxation exercise #1. This exercise acknowledges that you are in a zone of safety and can completely relax and let down your guard. Notice and then release tension throughout your body with each exhale.

Connect with your heartbeat and thus with your heart. As you notice your pulse, visualize its connection with your heart. When you feel the pulse, it's the pulse of blood flowing under your finger. That blood has come from your heart and ultimately will wind up back at your heart. Visualize this circulation and then your pulsing heart. Think of all your associations with the heart: it's the center and the source of life.

What other associations do you have? Say to yourself, "This is my heart. This is what has been 100 percent reliable my entire life, every single minute. It has never taken a single break. I can truly trust it." Imagine that this pulse you are now tuned in to is the representation of the rhythm of the universe within you. It is a reflection of the whole, residing inside you. Thus, right now you are tuning in to the universe—by tuning in to yourself. Focus on the feelings of love, either for yourself or for someone close to you. Imagine that each time you breathe in, you are expanding your heart and your experience of love. Now, meditate on this and feel yourself letting go—into your heart.

As you have worked the nine pillars and moved more and more onto The Path, you will have noticed a shift away from your primitive Gestalt patterns. The results include less fearfulness, greater joy and happiness, improved health, and greater success. You feel more in control of your life, with less anxiety or depression. The Path has taken you through a developmental process of personal growth and self-efficacy.

With diminished fear and anger, you are thinking more clearly and have less need to be hurtful to others. You are more connected to your loving center and your loving heart, and almost automatically, you send those "coherent" vibrations out into the world and to touch those around you. You are also noticing that people want to be around you more.

Moving The Path out beyond the nine pillars and deeper into your heart, as expressed in step three, you are generating fourth-level neurogenesis by connecting with the implicate order. To have a place inside that you can trust and always go to for stability—the calm in a storm—this will always stay with you. Do step three now.

STEP 3 *Connecting to the implicate order*

Imagine that as you deepen your connection with your heart, with your finger on your pulse, an amazing transformation begins to take place. I talked earlier in the book about the blueprint for growth set up by your primitive Gestalt pattern.

You are now connecting to the blueprint of the universe—what David Bohm referred to as the "implicate order." As you continue to deepen your personal process and let go, you connect more and more with this universal pattern.

DYING . . . IN ORDER TO LIVE FULLY

There have been times in my personal journey where I felt like I was on the threshold of a growth spurt, but my efforts stalled. Right at that point, it felt like I was giving up too much to move forward; it was too big a leap. In fact, it felt like moving forward would feel like dying. When I was finally able to make the leap—and it has happened more than once—I realized that a part of me did in fact die. Each of my growth spurts was accompanied by a letting go of some old messages and old ways of being. The good news is that it was nothing like what

I had feared. There was no pain, and I remained the same person, only at a new and more advanced level of development. Everything around me was clearer, and I carried myself with less fear. In fact, the biggest thing I let go of—the biggest thing that died—was a part of my fears.

The unknown, even when it's your own growth into a bigger and more mature self, can be experienced as scary and perhaps even feel like it will be some sort of death. But it will always turn out to be the best thing you ever did. You will never look back. Go to step four on The Path now.

STEP 4   *Heart coherence*

Focus on your heart by placing your hand over it. Feel and visualize its pulse, its beat. Focus on appreciation in your life and on projecting love out from your heart. Visualize this process facilitating the coherence of the rhythms of your body. Imagine these coherent rhythms bathing your body in healing energy.

Now, allow this rhythm to be projected out beyond the boundaries of your material body. Imagine this coherent wave and visualize it, however it might appear to you. The key is to imagine that the healthy, coherent rhythm you are generating moves out and surrounds your body.

As you feel and visualize this aura of coherent rhythm, imagine it repairing and healing the energy field that surrounds you. And finally, imagine this coherent aura projecting out into the universe.

MAKE THIS DEEPENING PROCESS AN ONGOING GOAL IN YOUR LIFE

The self-discovery process is sometimes referred to as peeling the layers off an onion. This is because your pattern goes very deep, and each time you engage in the healing process and peel another layer from your pattern, there it is again, but at a deeper level. With each layer, however, you do become healthier and more resilient. Also, as you go deeper, you open yourself to additional levels of existence and more healing energy that radiate out from the deepest part of yourself.

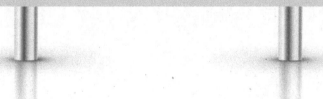

SIGNPOST

- You have identified something you were still holding on to and went through a process to facilitate letting go.
- You practiced a heart meditation.
- You are connecting to the blueprint of the universe.
- You are using your heart rhythm to heal the energy that you project out into the universe.

CHAPTER 18

STAYING ON THE PATH

'm frequently asked, "Will this process ever get easier?" "Will I always have to work this hard to get onto and to stay on The Path?" A very good question. It's like you have been going uphill all this time or climbing a mountain—when do you get to the top, or when will it feel like you are going downhill and coasting? I can answer this in three ways:

1. When you shift from your old habit patterns and old internal parent to new habits and an internal voice—your voice of wisdom—that support resilience as defined by my model, you will be over the hump.

2. When your center of gravity—the place where you come from, your home—has shifted from the primitive Gestalt spokesperson to a new, healthy internal voice, you will then be moving downhill.

3. When you embody The Path—when your muscle and sensing memories feel more comfortable on The Path; when you begin feeling and recognizing discomfort when you are off The

Path—you will have shifted into a new gear in life. It's like being able to detect true north without a compass.

One of the dichotomies we have been working with is the one between your old, internal parent—the one that's the lookout for your primitive Gestalt pattern—and a new, healthier internal parent. The new, healthier parent comes from a loving and accepting place. The more you have made the transition—the more fully you have nurtured and developed a healthy internal voice—the easier it will be to stay on The Path. And yes, it will then feel like going downhill. But this isn't to say you stop growing. Inviting challenges into your life and engaging the growing process are what maintain healthy epigenesis, neurogenesis, and regeneration. What you want to happen is that you engage in the growth process with the 9 Pillars of Resilience mastered.

What this looks like is that you aren't afraid to make a mistake, and you don't beat yourself up when you do make an error. You have a positive attitude and positive expectations. It means you don't deplete your energy by overreacting to a person or situation. And if you do, you immediately realize that you have unfinished business to address. Your openness to new ideas and ways of doing things stays with you, and you are able to be present a large percentage of the time. Most important, you feel good about and are accepting of yourself. Throughout this process, my intention has been to foster this development and this shift in your center of gravity.

Wake up! Being present in the moment is the gateway to The Path. Being present is like waking up from a dream. But here I'm referring to how we sleepwalk through life, only half aware and usually operating on automatic. So to stay on The Path requires some way for you to remember to wake up and be fully in the moment. In a previous chapter, you took a step on The Path with the "portal" exercise. This is where you remember yourself—that is, you notice, recognize, and witness yourself in that moment. You use each portal or doorway you walk through as a reminder to be aware of your existence. You are acknowledging yourself. Go to The Path now and do steps one, two, and three.

STEP 1 *Creating a reminder system*

Staying on The Path requires some sort of reminder system to wake you up when you begin to fall asleep.

Too easily the stresses of life, the media, and other distractions take you off The Path and back into habit patterns and unconsciousness. It's thus necessary to place cues or reminders someplace along your path. You have been creating affirmations that you read when you awaken, throughout the day, and before you go to sleep. Make sure you continue to utilize these messages on a daily basis for this purpose. Begin each day by declaring your intention to step onto The Path.

STEP 2 *Three-month reminder*

Whatever you use as your calendar or appointment book, go to a page three months from now and make a note to yourself that says, "Am I on The Path or off The Path?"

Add, "In what ways am I on The Path and how am I off The Path?" This will ensure that if you are off The Path and don't realize it, you will be reminded.

STEP 3 *Keeping the momentum going*

In three months, when you read the messages from step two, advance another three months in your calendar or appointment book and make the same note. And then continue this process every three months.

Here is what I would expect when you live your life on The Path: You will experience greater energy and greater recovery of energy after any exertion. You will experience fewer physical, emotional, and mental symptoms. In fact, being on The Path should result in your brain functioning at a higher level and maintaining higher levels of cognitive functioning into old age. You will have better blood flow to your brain, which will keep your brain functioning better and longer.

Getting to this point, you have experienced quite a lot of success. Think about how you have been able to either stay on The Path or get back onto The Path when you have strayed off it. To continue to achieve all that you want, you know that it's important to stay on The Path. You might also want to join my mailing list so you will receive any updates to this material, newsletters, and any future programs. You can do this by going to www.DrStephenSideroff.com.

The goal now is to make this into a lifelong healthy physical, emotional, and mental pattern. From this will come your most effective and successful performance and life. As noted in the introduction, my experience demonstrates that the challenges and stresses of life serve to take you off your desired course and out of these newly established patterns. There are two methods to staying on The Path:

1. Consciously maintaining the newly learned behaviors in order to continue establishing new, healthy brain pathways and habits, and

2. Maintaining a vision of a continually upward spiral of development, whereby you can return to the first pillar of resilience after completion of the book and go through the process again, but at a higher level—thus, the upward spiral. Do steps four, five, and six now.

STEP 4 | *Noting your success and accomplishments to this point*

Begin an assessment of your progress by retaking the Resilience Questionnaire that follows and comparing your current levels to where you started at the beginning of this program and in the middle of the program. Appreciate improvement along any of the 9 Pillars of Resilience. Take in these successes as emotional nourishment.

STEP 5 *What do you need to return to?*

Identify areas that need further development or that have been resistant to change. Return to those chapters and recommit to further work and progress.

STEP 6 *How have your symptoms improved?*

Retake the Symptom Checklist on page 373 and notice the improvement of your symptoms.

LAST WORDS

Having reached the last steps of The Path, it's now important for you to express appreciation and gratitude toward yourself for the heroic effort you have made in your own personal development. In fact, it's been a true hero's journey. You have done an amazing job. You have reshaped your behaviors and your brain. In the process, I'm sure you have also achieved success, along with improving relationships with others, yourself, and your community. Congratulations! Remember, The Path is always right there. If you fall off, as we all do, it's just steps away. Keep asking yourself the question, "Am I on The Path or off The Path?" Proceed once more to the Symptom Checklist and Path to Resilience and Success Questionnaire in the appendix on page 373. Note how you have grown through your journey on The Path.

SIGNPOST

- You are using cues to remind yourself of following The Path.
- You are using affirmations to help in your growth process.
- You have placed a reminder three months from now in your calendar or appointment book.
- You have retaken your Resilience Questionnaire and the Symptom Checklist and have noted your progress.
- You have taken note of areas still needing further development and are taking steps to follow up.

APPENDIX

Next to each symptom, please indicate your level using the following scale:
1 = Never, 2 = Rarely, 3 = Sometimes, 4 = Much of the time, 5 = Always

Physical		Behavioral		Emotional	
	Arthritis		Aggressiveness		Agitation
	Backaches		Compulsive eating		Anger
	Colitis		Daydreaming or escapist fantasies		Annoyance
	Constipation or hemorrhoids		Excessive throat clearing		Anxiety
	Diarrhea		Excessive use of alcohol to cope		Depression
	Fatigue, lack of energy		Forgetfulness		Despair
	Frequent colds		Insomnia, difficulty sleeping		Frustration
	Gas		Loss of appetite		Impatience
	Headaches		Poor posture		Inflexibility
	Heart disease		Quick temper		Irritability

Continues

Physical		Behavioral		Emotional
	High blood pressure		Racing thoughts	Loneliness
	Muscle tension		Repetitive behavior (e.g., tapping fingers)	Nervousness
	Muscle twitches or aches		Sighing	Powerlessness
	Rashes or itching		Teeth grinding	Rage
	Respiratory problems		Use of prescription or other drugs to cope	Sadness
	Stiffness in neck or shoulder			
	Stomachaches or tension			
	Ulcers			
Total Physical		**Total Behavioral**		**Total Emotional**

Category	Rate your level of stress from 1 (lowest) to 10 (highest)	Rate your ability to cope and handle from 1 to 10
Work stress		
Family stress		
Other personal stress		
Overall stress		

On average, how long does it take for you to fall asleep at night?

_____

On average, how many hours of sleep do you get at night?

_____

On average, how many hours do you work per week?

_____

Please answer each statement by circling the number that best describes your current views and life situation. Add your total score for each component and transfer this number to your Resilience Profile. Please answer to the best of your ability and as honestly as possible. This is for your own awareness. There are no right or wrong answers.

Statement	Not at all true			Very true
1. I feel good about myself; I like who I am.	0	1	2	3
2. I take care of myself; I exercise and eat right.	0	1	2	3
3. I have a hard time accepting compliments.	3	2	1	0
4. I am more apt to pick out what I did wrong rather than what I did right.	3	2	1	0
TOTAL SCORE: RELATIONSHIP WITH SELF				
5. I let people take advantage of me.	3	2	1	0
6. I have a good network of people in my life who want me to succeed.	0	1	2	3
7. It's hard for me to ask for help.	3	2	1	0
8. I have difficulty making friends.	3	2	1	0
TOTAL SCORE: RELATIONSHIP WITH OTHERS				
9. I find purpose in my life.	0	1	2	3
10. I am committed to giving service to a cause.	0	1	2	3
11. I believe in something greater than myself.	0	1	2	3
12. I want to make a difference in the world.	0	1	2	3
TOTAL SCORE: RELATIONSHIP WITH SOMETHING GREATER				

Continues

Statement	Not at all true			Very true
13. I am able to easily relax.	0	1	2	3
14. When stressed I recover quickly.	0	1	2	3
15. I have difficulty unwinding.	3	2	1	0
16. When I go to bed, it takes me a while to fall asleep, or I may toss and turn and not feel rested in the morning.	3	2	1	0
TOTAL SCORE: PHYSICAL BALANCE AND MASTERY				
17. I am not bothered by the judgments of others.	0	1	2	3
18. I don't dwell on mistakes.	0	1	2	3
19. When I wake up in the morning, I worry about what might happen during the day.	3	2	1	0
20. I am usually on the lookout for what can go wrong.	3	2	1	0
TOTAL SCORE: COGNITIVE BALANCE AND MASTERY				
21. I am aware of my feelings.	0	1	2	3
22. I am able to express my feelings.	0	1	2	3
23. I get impatient when others make mistakes, are slow, or don't understand things.	3	2	1	0
24. I overreact in certain situations.	3	2	1	0
25. I am able to let go of difficult feelings.	0	1	2	3
TOTAL SCORE: EMOTIONAL BALANCE AND MASTERY				
26. I don't notice details in my environment.	3	2	1	0
27. I am able to stay in the present.	0	1	2	3
28. I have confidence in myself.	0	1	2	3

Statement	Not at all true			Very true
29. I anticipate and take action instead of reacting to events.	0	1	2	3
30. I get distracted easily.	3	2	1	0
TOTAL SCORE: PRESENCE				
31. I am able to see the perspective of others.	0	1	2	3
32. I look for new experiences to learn from.	0	1	2	3
33. I have difficulty being flexible.	3	2	1	0
34. If my path is thwarted, I have difficulty improvising and adjusting to a more attainable goal.	3	2	1	0
TOTAL SCORE: FLEXIBILITY				
35. I do not let my fears stop me from taking action.	0	1	2	3
36. I have difficulty making important decisions.	3	2	1	0
37. I procrastinate before taking action.	3	2	1	0
38. I am able to be assertive to overcome an obstacle.	0	1	2	3
39. I have a strong will.	0	1	2	3
40. I have difficulty finishing what I start.	3	2	1	0
TOTAL SCORE: POWER				

THE PATH OF RESILIENCE PROFILE

	RELATIONSHIP			ORGANISMIC			PROCESS		
Optimal Functioning	12 11 10	12 11 10	12 11 10	12 11 10	12 11 10	15 14 13 12	15 14 13 12	12 11 10	18 17 16 15
Average Functioning	9 8 7	9 8 7	9 8 7	9 8 7	9 8 7	11 10 9 8	11 10 9 8	9 8 7	14 13 12 11 10
Borderline	6 5	6 5	6 5	6 5	6 5	7 6 5	7 6 5	6 5	9 8 7
Problem Area	4 3 2 1	4 3 2 1	4 3 2 1	4 3 2 1	4 3 2 1	4 3 2 1	4 3 2 1	4 3 2 1	6 5 4 3 2 1
	With Self	With Others	With Something Greater	Physiological	Cognitive	Emotional	Presence	Flexibility	Power

ACKNOWLEDGMENTS

There have been many people throughout my life who have been my teachers. I appreciate the following, some who, in their holding of friendships, gave me just the right support when it was needed, some who embodied one of my pillars, and those who have given me valuable feedback on my book and my ideas: Allen Darbonne, Hal Myers, Michael Sinel, Rob Lufkin, Eleanor Criswell, Butch Schuman, Hugh Baras, Paul Domitor, Neil Schneiderman, James McGaugh, Dalbir Bindra, Donald Hebb, Stephan Tobin, Murray Jarvik, Liana Mattulich, David Wellisch, Peter Levine, Jack Rosenberg, Barbara Manalis, Ron Klemp, Rabbi Benjamin Herson, Rabbi Judith HaLevy, Desiree Sideroff, Ali Sideroff, Sharon Sideroff, Kusala, Yahola Simms, Lorraine Sterman, Barry Sterman, George Von Bozzay, Phil Firestone, Jahan Stanizai, Armand Bytton, Steven Angel, Jim Gay, Bonnie Franklin, Eulogia Goree, Akil Goree, Laurie Levin, Jerry Levin, Ron Doctor, Kamyar Hedayat, Terry Kaplan, Lonnie Kaplan, Rebecca Tobias, Bob Edelman, Michael Lutsky, Lon Price, Beverly Spaulding, and Pittsburg Slim.

ABOUT THE AUTHOR

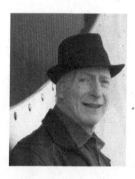 Dr. Stephen Sideroff is an internationally recognized psychologist, executive and medical consultant, and expert in resilience, longevity, optimal performance, addiction, neurofeedback, and mental health. He has published pioneering research in these fields. Dr. Sideroff's work focuses on the two most important and difficult modern issues we all face: stress and resilience, and achieving permanent change and transformation. His approach is focused not only on providing useful information, but presenting it in a way that produces change in the recipient.

Dr. Sideroff is an associate professor in the departments of psychiatry and biobehavioral sciences and rheumatology at UCLA's Geffen School of Medicine. He was the founder and former clinical director of the Stress Strategies program of UCLA Santa Monica Medical Center and former clinical director of Moonview Sanctuary's Treatment and Optimal Performance Center. He has helped establish innovative training and treatment approaches in optimal functioning, mind-body medicine in the US, China, and Europe, and hosted summits on longevity, resilience and leadership. His innovative model of resilience presented to organizations and individuals has been hailed as "a true Bible for living in balance and spirituality." In his free time, Dr. Sideroff enjoys family, mountain biking and playing the saxophone.